Early Modern History: Society and Culture

General Editors: **Rab Houston**, Professor of Early Modern History, University of St Andrews, Scotland and **Edward Muir**, Professor of History, Northwestern University, Illinois

This series encompasses all aspects of early modern international history from 1400 to *c*.1800. The editors seek fresh and adventurous monographs, especially those with a comparative and theoretical approach, from both new and established scholars.

Titles include:

Robert C. Davis
CHRISTIAN SLAVES, MUSLIM MASTERS
White Slavery in the Mediterranean, the Barbary Coast, and Italy, 1500–1800

Rudolf Dekker
CHILDHOOD, MEMORY AND AUTOBIOGRAPHY IN HOLLAND
From the Golden Age to Romanticism

Caroline Dodds Pennock
BONDS OF BLOOD
Gender, Lifecycle and Sacrifice in Aztec Culture

Steve Hindle
THE STATE AND SOCIAL CHANGE IN EARLY MODERN ENGLAND, 1550–1640

Katharine Hodgkin
MADNESS IN SEVENTEENTH CENTURY AUTOBIOGRAPHY

Craig M. Koslofsky
THE REFORMATION OF THE DEAD
Death and Ritual in Early Modern Germany, 1450–1700

Beat Kümin
DRINKING MATTERS
Public Houses and Social Exchange in Early Modern Central Europe

John Jeffries Martin
MYTHS OF RENAISSANCE INDIVIDUALISM

A. Lynn Martin
ALCOHOL, SEX AND GENDER IN LATE MEDIEVAL AND EARLY MODERN EUROPE

Laura J. McGough
GENDER, SEXUALITY, AND SYPHILIS IN EARLY MODERN VENICE
The Disease that Came to Stay

Samantha A. Meigs
THE REFORMATIONS IN IRELAND
Tradition and Confessionalism, 1400–1690

Craig Muldrew
THE ECONOMY OF OBLIGATION
The Culture of Credit and Social Relations in Early Modern England

Niall Ó Ciosáin
PRINT AND POPULAR CULTURE IN IRELAND, 1750–1850

H. Eric R. Olsen
THE CALABRIAN CHARLATAN, 1598–1603
Messianic Nationalism in Early Modern Europe

Thomas Max Safley
MATHEUS MILLER'S MEMOIR
A Merchant's Life in the Seventeenth Century

Clodagh Tait
DEATH, BURIAL AND COMMEMORATION IN IRELAND, 1550–1650

Richard W. Unger
SHIPS ON MAPS
Pictures of Power in Renaissance Europe

Johan Verberckmoes
LAUGHTER, JESTBOOKS AND SOCIETY IN THE SPANISH NETHERLANDS

Claire Walker
GENDER AND POLITICS IN EARLY MODERN EUROPE
English Convents in France and the Low Countries

Johannes C. Wolfart
RELIGION, GOVERNMENT AND POLITICAL CULTURE IN EARLY MODERN
GERMANY
Lindau, 1520–1628

Forthcoming title:

Caroline Dodds
LIVING WITH SACRIFICE

Early Modern History: Society and Culture
Series Standing Order ISBN 978–0–333–71194–1 (Hardback)
978–0–333–80320–2 (Paperback)
(*outside North America only*)

You can receive future titles in this series as they are published by placing a stand-ing order. Please contact your bookseller or, in case of difficulty, write to us at the address below with your name and address, the title of the series and the ISBN quoted above.

Customer Services Department, Macmillan Distribution Ltd, Houndmills, Basingstoke, Hampshire RG21 6XS, England

Gender, Sexuality, and Syphilis in Early Modern Venice

The Disease that Came to Stay

Laura J. McGough
Lecturer, Department of Population, Family, and Reproductive Health, School of Public Health, University of Ghana

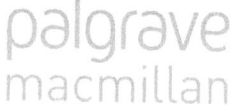

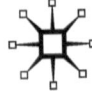
First published 2011 by
PALGRAVE MACMILLAN

Palgrave Macmillan in the UK is an imprint of Macmillan Publishers Limited,
registered in England, company number 785998, of Houndmills, Basingstoke,
Hampshire RG21 6XS.

Palgrave Macmillan in the US is a division of St Martin's Press LLC,
175 Fifth Avenue, New York, NY 10010.

Palgrave Macmillan is the global academic imprint of the above companies
and has companies and representatives throughout the world.

Palgrave® and Macmillan® are registered trademarks in the United States,
the United Kingdom, Europe and other countries.

ISBN 978–0–230–25292–9   hardback

This book is printed on paper suitable for recycling and made from fully
managed and sustained forest sources. Logging, pulping and manufacturing
processes are expected to conform to the environmental regulations of the
country of origin.

A catalogue record for this book is available from the British Library.

A catalog record for this book is available from the Library of Congress.

10   9   8   7   6   5   4   3   2   1
20   19   18   17   16   15   14   13   12   11

Transferred to Digital Printing in 2014

For Olaf

Contents

List of Figures, Tables, and Charts

Figures

Tables

Charts

Acknowledgments

As this book attempts to bridge disciplines, I have been fortunate to receive advice and assistance from a variety of people from different backgrounds. More than a decade ago, I became interested in a convent for "repentant prostitutes" (few of whom were actually prostitutes, as it turns out) and how gender, sexuality, and religion intersected in this institution. The convent originated in a hospital for "French disease" (commonly but problematically translated as syphilis) patients. Later I was intrigued by how and why this institution formed part of a response to disease. In order to answer this question, I sought help from within and beyond the field of history: from physicians, epidemiologists, literary scholars, and art historians. Eventually, my interest in disease itself and its relationship to the larger society as it becomes endemic overtook some of my earlier interests.

First I owe thanks to those who introduced me to the world of Venetian and Italian history: especially Ed Muir, who first advised me to go to Venice and served as my dissertation adviser at Northwestern University. Chris Friedrichs at the University of British Columbia had earlier inspired an interest in early modern European history with his lively lectures. Thanks to the community of scholars of Venice, especially Guido Ruggiero, Jutta Sperling, Stanley Chojnacki, Anne Jacobson Schutte, Joanne Ferraro, Francesca Trivellato, Federico Barbierato, Chiara Vazzoler, Maria Fusaro, Monica Chojnacka, Liz Horodowich, Holly Hurlburt, and Karl Appuhn. A Fulbright fellowship enabled me to do my initial research, while the Gladys Krieble Delmas Foundation supported subsequent research to study gender and patterns of disease.

A 2001 NEH Summer Institute, led by Al Rabil, introduced me to other scholars within the humanities whose advice has been appreciated, especially Suzanne Magnanini.

Jonathan Zenilman opened doors for me and provided opportunities seldom available to historians. He introduced me to a lively group of scientists and clinicians working on sexually transmitted diseases at Johns Hopkins University and served as my mentor for a postdoctoral fellowship in STD prevention at both the Centers for Disease Control and Prevention (CDC) and Johns Hopkins (the ATPM fellowship). For their stimulating conversations on STDs, thanks to Ann Rompalo, Emily Erbelding, Tom Quinn, David Celentano, Ron Gray, Khalil Ghanem,

Rebecca Brotman, Rachel Anita Weber, Hope Johnson, and the Hopkins STD community; thanks to Sevgi Aral and John Douglas at the CDC in Atlanta, where I spent four months working with a team of scientists at the Behavioral Interventions Branch; and thanks to King Holmes, the "king" of current STD studies in the US for making time for me to interview him. During my postdoctoral fellowship, Randy Packard allowed me to use office space at the Institute for the History of Medicine and to participate in weekly seminars, as well as offered encouragement.

My current institutional home is the University of Ghana. I owe thanks especially to Kofi Baku for keeping my teaching load manageable while I was finishing this manuscript. Thanks also to Professor C. N. B. Tagoe, the former Vice Chancellor of the University of Ghana, and Fred Binka, Dean of the School of Public Health, for their appreciation of how historians can contribute to the field of public health.

The librarians and archivists at a number of institutions have been helpful, including the National Library of Medicine in Bethesda, the History of Medicine library at Johns Hopkins University, the Folger Library in Washington DC, the Marciana library in Venice, the state archives of Venice, the IRE library on the Giudecca, and the Vatican archive.

A number of people read and commented on chapters or entire drafts of this manuscript. Thanks to Jon Arrizabalaga, Kevin Siena, David Gentilcore, Mike Bailey, Francesca Trivellato, Stephan Miescher, the members of the Department of the History of Medicine at Johns Hopkins University, Jim Bono, and the participants in the 2003–4 Folger Library Colloquium that he organized on the topic, "Imagining Nature." Special thanks to the series editors of Palgrave Macmillan, Ed Muir and Rab Houston, and to Ruth Ireland for her editorial assistance. Any errors are my responsibility.

My family and friends have provided emotional support for a long time. Thanks to my father, Ed McGough and his wife Sharon, for their knowledge of and interest in all things medical. Thanks to my mother, Rosanne Kaufmann and her husband Martin, for their passion for all things Italian. Thanks to friends and family for their acts of encouragement and support, especially Rebecca Shereikis, Jeff McGough, Julie McFarland, Simon Baatz, Michelle Scott, Nat Amarteifio, Lauren Kula, Dan Todes, Madalyn McGough, Austin Riter, Giulia Barrera, Abena Osseo-Asare, and Trish Graham. Thanks above all to my husband, Olaf Kula, to whom this book is dedicated and whose intellectual curiosity and emotional support made this book possible.

Introduction

Beginning with the French invasion of Naples and spreading to involve three other European countries in a contest to control the Italian peninsula, the Italian Wars (1494–1530) brought lasting changes to the region. As a result of these wars, Milan and Naples fell under direct Spanish rule; the "eternal city" of Rome was sacked and took decades to recover its role as a leading center of patronage, arts, and culture; Florence's last republican government collapsed, leaving Venice as the only major city-state with a republican form of government. Although the city-states did recover and Rome in particular regained its authority, the Wars nonetheless brought about a decline in the prestige and independence of the Italian peninsula.[1] Finally, the Wars brought epidemic disease, including a disease that became associated with the invading army's destructiveness.

In Venice and throughout Italy, military leaders and army physicians reported a new disease which became popularly known as the "French disease" (often considered to be syphilis) because of its appearance after the French invasion of Naples.[2] Field reports from Venice's army physician Alessandro Benedetti included speculation that the invading French army in their haste ate poorly cooked pork, a possible cause of the new disease, a suggestion that borrowed from concepts of pollution and contamination.[3] Back at home, the prolific Venetian diarist Marin Sanuto duly noted any news he received about this illness in his lengthy entries on the war's progress. In 1498 and 1499, for example, Sanuto reported the French disease as he did any other illness, with no apparent sense of stigma or moral opprobrium. "*Item*, that Paulo Vitelli has a lot of the French disease." And Dom. Alvosio Valaresso had the French disease; he wanted to give money to the company, saying that he had no pay and was desperate.[4]

Concern grew as the disease impaired Venetian military strength. In 1499, for example, he reported that a Venetian galley at Corfu was unable to set sail because the crew was infected with the French disease.[5] In Florence, popular preacher Girolamo Savonarola quickly described the new disease in moral terms, as a scourge inflicted by God on the Florentines as punishment for their sins.[6] Early responses thereby included a mix of the practical, the speculative, and the moral; explanations of disease simultaneously invoked natural processes as well as signaled moral breakdown and the potential violation of social taboos. As this apparently new disease spread, it generated widespread controversy, debates, and anxiety among contemporaries. Some of the controversy, especially about the disease's origins and clinical manifestations, continues to this day. Modern scholars continue to discuss whether the French disease was the same as venereal syphilis, and whether the disease originated in the New World and was brought to Europe. These questions will be briefly addressed later in this chapter.

As interesting as the early years of the French disease epidemic were, they have captured the majority of scholarly attention, while the period from the mid-sixteenth century onwards has been relatively neglected. This book tackles this critical period and the issues that arise: how society responded to this disease once it was no longer new; what happened after the disease became widely regarded as sexually transmitted and curable; and the disease's relationship to culture, society, sexuality, and perceptions of stigma and morality during this period. *Gender, Sexuality, and Syphilis in Early Modern Venice* examines the social, cultural, and institutional processes in which the French disease became established as an endemic disease in early modern Venice during the sixteenth and seventeenth centuries. My principal focus is not about the literal distribution of disease within Venice's population, although I do discuss what can be known about disease distribution based on historical sources. Therefore, it is not primarily a study in historical epidemiology. Instead, it is a cultural and social history of disease.

The transition from epidemic to endemic disease needs to be understood as not only an epidemiological transition, but also as a social, cultural, and institutional process. The transition from epidemic to endemic disease meant that Venice's social and sexual networks produced a pattern that made the disease relatively common and widely distributed across neighborhoods, social class, and occupation, as well as evenly balanced between men and women. As an endemic disease, the French disease became embedded in Venice's cultural myths and in its network of charitable institutions and health care. Endemic diseases require careful attention to the social and cultural processes that sustain and reproduce diseases within populations, as well as to the ways in which societies construct a disease as epidemic, and therefore worthy of extraordinary attention, or endemic, and therefore "normal" and more easily ignored. Carefully inscribed within Venetian patterns of social, cultural, and institutional responses to disease, the French disease no longer demanded special attention by the late sixteenth century until a new crisis occurred during the eighteenth century.

Early modern Venetians, educated or not, did not use the word "endemic" to describe their understanding of the French disease. I have chosen to use the modern word "endemic" for two reasons: first and most importantly, in order to synthesize and reconstruct the ways in which Venetian responses to the French disease had changed by the late sixteenth century; and secondly to invite comparisons with various endemic diseases in different time periods and contexts. The word endemic enables modern readers to see a historical transition that may not have been absolutely clear to the people living through it. One job of the historian is to discern larger patterns and major transitions that are not readily evident to people at the time.

Venetian responses to the French disease combined moral and physical care of patients, while simultaneously integrating these responses into Venice's system of gender norms. For example, I will show how Venice's network of female asylums formed part of the system of French disease prevention and care. Venetian political and ecclesiastical authorities singled out females as potential sources of infection and responded in two ways. If they had not yet lost their virginity, they were reintegrated into society in ways that did not challenge gender norms, as marriageable young adult women enclosed within a Catholic institution until the day they married; or, if they had lost their virginity, they were removed from society in socially accepted ways, as repentant Magdalenes who became nuns. This gendered system helped "normalize" the French disease by integrating its victims within socially accepted roles.

Modern readers may find themselves wondering whether this historical study offers any insights into the problems we face now, especially with the pandemic of HIV/AIDS and the ongoing struggles with sexually transmitted diseases, some of which—human papilloma virus, chlamydia, herpes, to name just a few—have only been identified within the last two or three decades but whose impact is widespread and significant. It is certainly no accident that I am writing on this topic as the HIV/AIDS pandemic will soon move into its fourth decade and is now regarded as an endemic disease in many countries, especially in sub-Saharan Africa, where I currently live and work. I have spent a significant part of my professional life working on HIV/AIDS prevention, treatment, and care, and confronted how intransigent diseases can become within populations once they are regarded as "normal," inevitable, or confined to a socially "deviant" population. This book therefore includes an afterword with a few observations on how historical studies can help inform our response to current struggles against HIV/AIDS and other diseases, especially neglected endemic ones.

More than 30 years ago, William McNeill paved the way for the study of how epidemic diseases become "domesticated," as he put it (or endemic), especially in the Mongol invasion of Europe and the European conquest of the New World. The domestication of epidemic diseases such as yellow fever depended on the establishment of the mosquito species *Aedes aegypti*, which served as a vector, into the ecology of the New World, which apparently first occurred in sufficient numbers to cause an epidemic in 1648. Afterwards, epidemics occurred with regular frequency, indicating that the disease had become "domesticated" or endemic.[7] McNeill does not go into any detail about the processes by which the French disease (he uses the term 'syphilis') became domesticated, probably because he was writing before the explosion of research into historical patterns of sexuality and sexual behavior. This book fills in the gaps, examining the "domestication" of disease not only as a biological process, but also as a social, cultural, and institutional process.

Gender, Sexuality, and Syphilis in Early Modern Venice builds upon major contributions to the study of the French disease in early modern Europe, as well as upon the sizeable and growing body of literature on the social construction of illness and concepts from the medical anthropology of HIV/AIDS.[8] Jon Arrizabalaga, John Henderson, and Roger French have described part of this process of transition from epidemic to "endemic" disease through their careful study of medical and institutional responses to the French disease, although they have avoided the use of modern scientific terms.[9] In particular, two crucial intellectual transitions occurred as a result of Europeans' experience with the French disease. First, European physicians believed that they had discovered effective therapies for the French disease, including guaiacum and mercury. Controversy raged over which therapies were most effective, but the disease had moved from the category of incurable to curable.

Second, European physicians reached a consensus that diseases were a kind of specific entity. This ontological idea of disease coexisted and overlapped with an older tradition, based on Hippocratic/Galenic medicine, of disease as an imbalance of fluids within the body brought about by individual behavior, climate changes, or some combination of circumstances that upset a body's internal balance. The ontological view of disease had important implications.[10] As specific entities, diseases thereby had histories. According to many early modern physicians, the French disease had arrived in Europe in the late fifteenth century as a young disease, full of strength, and had by the mid-sixteenth century grown old, weakened, and was more easily controlled through medications. Although some modern historians have been tempted to read these sixteenth-century accounts of the disease's life cycle quite literally as evidence that the disease became less virulent, the sources themselves suggest a change in European perceptions of disease, not necessarily a change in the disease itself; yet it is possible that both perceptions and the disease itself underwent a transformation.[11]

By the mid-sixteenth century, physicians' perception that they were facing an old, curable disease helps explain why they reacted without alarm to the continued presence of the French disease. This transition from "young" epidemic disease to "weak" endemic disease is crucial in understanding how and why certain patients suffered stigma from the French disease while others suffered relatively little stigma or even escaped it altogether. Medical care became routine for French disease cases, with a variety of therapies available for the first-time sufferer as well as the return patient. Cases that did not respond to therapy disrupted the routine management of the sick. The process of stigmatization itself thereby underwent change, as patients who suffered from apparently incurable cases bore the brunt of stigma from the mid-sixteenth century onwards, in contrast to the earlier period. Physicians and the public blamed patients, not the failure of medical therapies, for incurable cases of French disease; allegedly "promiscuous" women and "dissolute" men were particular targets because they represented social and moral disorder as well as physical contagion.

This study extends recent work in the cultural history of the French disease to show how Europeans began to incorporate this disease into their local and national mythologies and icons, defined as part of a process of making the disease "endemic" at the cultural level. Historians and literary theorists have already shown how perception of the French disease changed between the late fifteenth to the mid-sixteenth centuries. Foa has argued that initial responses to the epidemic borrowed heavily from the iconography of leprosy, as Europeans sought ways to make the unfamiliar disease more familiar.[12] By the mid-sixteenth century, Europeans incorporated the French disease into their own cultural myths, stories, and images, and thereby the disease became endemic to European cultures. Certain themes were virtually universal among Europeans of the early modern period: the oft-noted tendency to blame foreigners for disease, for example, and hence the name the "French disease" or the "Neapolitan disease."[13]

Other themes, while perhaps discernible throughout Europe, acquired a greater cultural importance in specific geographic areas because of literary and cultural traditions or social practices specific to each area. In Venice, the public associated the French disease with extremely beautiful "promiscuous" women and with undisciplined or dissolute men. In a city-state often represented as a beautiful woman and continually threatened by war with the Turks during the sixteenth century, a woman's alluring beauty could be a troubling image to Venetians, especially when coupled with an undisciplined military force tasked with defending its receding borders. The trope of the beautiful, dangerous woman was already a familiar one to Venetians for a variety of reasons. Beautiful women from a lower social class represented a potential threat to Venice's nobility, the most socially exclusive nobility in Europe and least open to marriage to non-noble women. Passion and sexual attraction were potentially disruptive forces that could threaten the ruling classes' social cohesion; these anxieties easily found expression in the trope of a beautiful but diseased woman's body.[14] In Tuscany, the French disease became associated with the dangers of sodomy to the body politic, an already-established trope and political preoccupation since well before the late fifteenth-century epidemic.[15] In early modern England, the French disease became associated with a variety of practices that brought moral condemnation from contemporaries, including the importation of silk, satin and velvet textiles—luxuries, which allegedly weakened England's moral fabric and made English people more susceptible to moral vice and disease.[16] Although each narrative of danger varies from region to region in Europe, the common theme is that the French disease became incorporated into different tropes of "danger" to the body politic and society. Venice therefore is illustrative of a more general process—that is, the incorporation of the French disease into cultural myths and literary tropes—taking place throughout Europe, although the specifics are different in each location.[17]

This book draws on recent work about institutional responses to the French disease. Kevin Siena has shown how common it was for French disease patients to receive treatment from various kinds of institutions in early modern London, notably the city's extensive network of workhouse infirmaries. Although workhouses were not designed to provide medical treatment for the poor but rather to discipline the poor through a strict regimen of forced labor, they nonetheless became the last resort for medical care for London's impoverished inhabitants, with French disease patients constituting as much as 70 percent of one workhouse's inmates in the late eighteenth century.[18] Access to institutional care was fractured along London's class and gender divides, with men and the wealthy having greater access to private physicians, working-class men having greater access to hospital care than working-class women, and finally a concentration of impoverished women in the workhouse infirmaries, the least desirable form of care because patients were not allowed bed rest or confidential treatment.[19]

Response to the French disease was also embedded within Venice's network of charitable institutions. These institutions, especially Venice's female asylums, bore a heavy burden of providing care to current or former French disease patients. Some institutions, such as the hospital for the Incurables and a convent for repentant *meretrici* (promiscuous women), were established as part of a response to the French disease. The sixteenth century witnessed an enormous growth in the number of charitable institutions, fuelled by the religious reform movements of the late fifteenth and early sixteenth centuries as well as by the perceived need to provide care for the sick. Venice's institutions represented a gendered response to disease. For the prevention and control of the French disease, females were placed in one of several institutions: the Zitelle, an enclosed, residential institution designed to prepare poor girls for marriage or the convent and thereby prevent them from being "debauched" at a young age; the Casa del Soccorso, a temporary shelter for prostitutes, promiscuous women, and abused wives; the above-mentioned Convertite, a convent for repentant *meretrici*; or during the eighteenth century, the *Penitenti*, another refuge for "promiscuous" women.[20] While previous scholars have mentioned the origins of these institutions within hospitals that primarily treated French disease patients,[21] this study examines the origin and development of these institutions within Venice's gendered perceptions of the French disease. Although, like London's workhouses, these female asylums played multiple roles and never exclusively functioned in order to care for French disease patients, they nonetheless were a crucial part of Venice's overall strategy to control the French disease.

This study makes three important contributions to the history of early modern medicine, sexuality, culture, and society. First, it draws attention to the ways in which early modern Venetians' experiences of and responses to the French disease had changed by the mid-sixteenth century as the disease became "endemic" in the broadest possible sense: that is, embedded within the culture, within social patterns of sexuality and reproduction, and within medical and institutional care. This book thereby encourages scholars to see the transition from epidemic to endemic disease not just as a biological or epidemiological process, but rather as a process that involves culture, social relations, politics, and institutions. Examining responses to diseases as a cultural, social, political, and institutional process is a common approach in medical anthropology and history of medicine, but most of this attention has focused on epidemic or chronic disease in a particular society,[22] not on the cultural, social, and institutional processes themselves as crucial in the transition from epidemic to endemic disease.[23] In the case of the French disease, some scholars have described certain aspects of change in response to the disease during the sixteenth century, especially changes in medical theory and cultural myths, but they have not identified these changes as part of a broader transition from epidemic to endemic disease.[24] This study explains how "visible," epidemic diseases can become "invisible" over time, despite their continued costs in human suffering, pain, and disfigurement.[25]

Second, this study analyzes the history of the French disease through the perspective of gender, an analysis that is largely missing in works on the early modern period.[26] Gender is critical to understanding how early modern Venetians perceived and responded to the French disease. Perceptions of both masculinity and femininity informed the way Venetians responded to disease: for men, acquisition of the French disease could serve as a badge of honor, indicating successful conquest on the sexual battlefield; for women, however, the disease was usually shameful. These gender norms influenced sexual behavior and impaired women's ability to seek medical care openly. Furthermore, charitable institutions themselves were divided by gender: only girls and women were placed in institutions to encourage their repentance or to prevent them from acquiring sexual experience and, in consequence, the French disease. Moral and gendered perceptions of the French disease built on and reinforced social prejudices and hierarchies, exacerbated inequalities between men and women by offering different types and quality of medical and institutional care, and helped create and sustain support for the institutionalization of certain categories of women, especially unmarried beautiful women and girls.

Third, I situate the history of the French disease within the history of sexuality. Scholars have understandably been reluctant to make claims about which sexual practices have contributed to the spread of disease historically. Nonetheless, because the disease was regarded as primarily transmitted through sexual activity during this period, it is not anachronistic to place the disease within the context of early modern sexual relations. Although the study of early modern sexuality has largely focused on discursive practices rather than on empirical behavior,[27] there is nonetheless a great deal to be learned about behavior from discursive practices, as demonstrated by a wide range of historians working on criminal records and other materials.[28] In particular, this book draws attention to the context in which sexual relations took place in early modern Venice: sexual violence that was unofficially tolerated; laws and policies that simultaneously restricted women's access to financial resources while requiring that she bring a dowry to marriage, thereby fostering conditions that encouraged the exchange of sex for survival; customs and inheritance practices that restricted noblemen's ability to marry in order to preserve family wealth while tacitly accepting noblemen's multiple sexual partnerships; seasonal and periodic labor migration of individuals between Venice and the mainland; and chronic economic and political insecurity. These "structural" factors influenced but did not determine human sexual behavior.[29]

There have been surprisingly few studies of the French disease or even of modern venereal syphilis that have examined the broader context of sexual relations. Instead, scholars have focused on the repression of prostitution.[30] Ironically, however, works that focus on prostitution alone may have inadvertently reinforced rather than challenged the idea that to control prostitution is to control sexually transmitted diseases. Physicians and public health reformers therefore have to keep relearning the same message over and over again: the control of prostitution alone does not eliminate disease transmission, because disease can be transmitted through a variety of sexual activities, paid or unpaid.[31]

The French disease: Problems of interpretation

Several theoretical and methodological questions need to be raised about how to approach the history of disease and sexuality and about source materials. Although the French disease has often been equated with the modern disease known as syphilis, there are several problems with this identification. First, during the fifteenth century, diseases were identified according to a set of symptoms, not an underlying, specific causative agent, such as the spirochete *treponema pallidum*, identified as the causative agent for syphilis that could be detected through the Wasserman test in the early twentieth century. The way physicians and patients have understood disease before and after the laboratory revolution is fundamentally different: to call the disease syphilis runs the risk of importing the whole set of modern connotations that accompany the disease.[32] Chapter 3 describes how early modern physicians reached a diagnosis through a combination of observation of ongoing symptoms and patient history; physicians believed that diseases resulted from underlying imbalances in body fluids, which could change over time and create a different set of symptoms. Furthermore, to try to understand past therapeutic practices, patients' experiences of illness, or the physician–patient relationship without understanding how different diseases were defined and conceptualized is a nearly impossible task.[33]

Second, early modern physicians did not distinguish between syphilis and gonorrhea, thereby making it possible that cases of the French disease referred to either one of these modern diseases, or perhaps a different disease altogether. It is therefore misleading to use the term 'syphilis', because, according to our modern understanding, the disease may have been gonorrhea or something else. My use of the word endemic is not potentially misleading in the way that the word syphilis is. Finally, this disease was typically diagnosed as the "French disease," often with the Latin name "morbus gallicus" rather than the term 'syphilis'. Although the word 'syphilis' was first used in 1530 by Girolamo Fracastoro in his epic poem, the word syphilis was seldom used clinically.[34] The name "the French disease" itself perfectly illustrates the problems presented in interpreting the historical evidence. Named after the invader, the French disease evoked a dual set of intertwined reactions: to wartime and ultimate military defeat, as well as to the disease itself. The 1490s were a period of intense religious fervor, as popular preachers such as Girolamo Savonarola anticipated the second coming of Christ in the year 1500 and God's punishment of sin. It was easy to see the French army, and subsequent disease, famine, and destruction, as divine punishment.[35] With skin lesions figuring prominently as one of the symptoms of the new French disease, the public was quick to see parallels with the afflictions of the biblical Job, whose faith was tested by God with the appearance of boils on his skin.[36] Whether or not the disease was associated with sexuality, it could still represent God's punishment, much as Job, an innocent man, was tested by God. Use of the term 'the French disease' thereby reminds readers of the specific connotations associated with the disease, connotations that are lost with the term 'syphilis.' I use the term 'syphilis' in the title to communicate with readers who may not be familiar with the context of early modern Italy, but the rest of the book will use the term 'the French disease.'

The first European French disease epidemic occurred in the context of wartime, during the French invasion of Italy in 1494 and the Spanish defense of Naples. Although the French army retreated, it did not do so quickly. At the Battle of Fornovo in 1495, the French army faced the combined forces of the Holy Roman Empire, the Spanish, several Italian city-states, including the papacy and the republics of Milan and Venice, with mercenary soldiers hired from throughout Europe. The other major European powers remained to vie for control of the Italian peninsula. The French returned in 1508 in a war of constantly shifting alliances between the major powers of Europe and the Italian city-states, which shifted alliances among themselves. Meanwhile, these armies continued to rely on mercenary soldiers.[37] The Italian Wars' long duration (until 1530) meant that foreign soldiers remained on Italian soil long enough to form short- and long-term sexual relationships with local women, not to mention war's usual impact on rape and prostitution. Venetian soldiers, who often came from the Holy Roman Empire, were billeted in towns and intermarried with the local population.[38] Furthermore, the disruptions of war brought famine and epidemics of a variety of diseases, including numerous "fevers" in addition to the French disease. It is important to underscore the significance of this war, which included the violent sacking of the city of Rome in 1527, as the context in which this epidemic took place. Too much of the literature on the historical origins of syphilis have described only the initial battle, but not the subsequent war. The creation of new sexual relationships, consensual or forced, temporary or long-term, as a result of the war and occupation helps explain why an epidemic was first identified on the Italian peninsula, in addition to the fact that the Italian city-states were the only part of Europe that possessed a rudimentary disease surveillance system.

Many scholars have primarily been interested in where this new disease originated, rather than in where it first assumed epidemic form. One continuing controversy is whether the disease originated in the New World and was brought back to Europe via Columbus's ships or already existed in other parts of Europe. It is not my intention to rehearse the various hypotheses here, which I and others have done elsewhere.[39] In fact, the ultimate geographical origins of the late fifteenth-century French disease epidemic—from the New World via Columbus and his sailors, or from northern Europe—are difficult to establish with certainty from present evidence. A recent study of DNA evidence is highly suggestive that the disease probably originated in the New World, but not yet definitive.[40] We can, however, surmise that the disease was probably new to a localized region, specifically where the first reports of an epidemic originated on the Italian peninsula. Although many of Columbus's sailors did become sick and some researchers have argued that the illness must have been syphilis based on symptoms described as "buboes," Spanish physicians did not refer to a new disease, or mention the French disease by name, until the early sixteenth century, after the epidemic had broken out on the Italian peninsula.[41]

The Italian city-states were the first to develop permanent public health offices and track causes of death, perhaps part of the reason that reports of a "new" disease first emerged from that region.[42] It is not possible to evaluate records from England or any other part of Europe during this period to ascertain whether the disease was new to that region. Mortality records, which had been carefully maintained in Milan since 1452 to track plague epidemics, do provide evidence that the disease was new at least to the Italian peninsula and therefore represented an epidemic. Milanese physicians had diagnosed leprosy as a cause of death since 1452, while the French disease represented a new disease category since 1503.[43] Therefore, the French disease epidemic was not merely an artifact of reporting errors based on inability to distinguish between the two diseases, as has been suggested.[44] In northern and central Italy, the disease was apparently new.

Although never as virulent and acute as plague, the French disease presented problems of its own, perhaps precisely because people often survived for years with this chronic disease rather than perish within days. Too sick to work, people survived by begging alms on the street. During the 1530s, Venetians regarded the presence of these street beggars as a double threat: to the physical as well as the moral health of the entire city.[45] Public response to disease combined moral and physical reform. Since God's punishment could descend on an entire city in the form of illness, Venetians during the early sixteenth century thought it was necessary to protect the entire city as a whole from the sins of the few by sending a small group of women to a convent dedicated to Mary Magdalene.

Venice's response to the French disease contained elements that were common to other Italian cities as well as elements that were unique to Venice. Hospitals and female asylums were part of a broader Catholic wave of institution building during the sixteenth century that encompassed the entire peninsula. Medical ideas and practices also spread widely throughout the Italian peninsula. Medical and institutional responses to the French disease were therefore not unique to Venice, but part of a wider Italian pattern. Cultural responses to the disease, as well as patterns of social and sexual networks, are much more specific to Venice. Each city-state seemed to have its own dominant tropes in representing the French disease, although there were common themes here as well, such as fear of foreigners. Venice's elite marriage practices differed from other cities in that it was much more difficult for a Venetian nobleman to marry than for some other Italian nobleman, leading to widespread liaisons with women of other social classes. In addition, as icon and as historical figure, Venice's courtesans played a much more visible, even public, role than in other Italian cities, with the exception of Rome. Although some of this study describes practices and ideas unique to Venice, I hope that this book will nonetheless be useful to scholars of other times and places by highlighting the role of cultural, social, and institutional processes in the transition from epidemic to endemic disease. Although the specifics of these processes will vary across space and time, it is nonetheless important to identify these processes and how they function in particular environments.

I chose Venice because of the advantages it offers in studying cultural, social and institutional responses to the French disease during the sixteenth and seventeenth centuries. As one of Europe's largest cities, Venice possessed both medical and public health expertise, with the nearby University of Padua's renowned medical faculty, as well as an organized public health office that left a paper trail for future historians. In addition, Venice is one of the few Italian cities in which records of the Inquisition trials are available for scholars; the trials are a rich, complex source of popular attitudes towards health and healing, as well as a source of information about sexuality. Because they are products of a legal process, they are also problematic sources which require careful attention to the ways in which witnesses' testimonies were shaped by the context of the trial and of legal procedures.[46] I have used a variety of other sources, including mortality records, the records of the female asylums, various court records relating to sexuality, Health Office records, and printed medical books aimed at a general audience. Because this study focuses on social, cultural, and institutional responses to disease rather than debates within the medical community about disease, I have restricted my sources to the vernacular medical writings. As the book proceeds, I will explain the strengths and limitations of these sources related to the particular issues under discussion.

The plan of the book is the following. In Chapter 1, I argue that the French disease became an endemic disease in early modern Venice in the literal sense of the word endemic: it was widely and evenly distributed throughout the population according to gender, neighborhood, and even social class and presented a consistent number of cases each year. Based on mortality data gathered for 24 years during the late sixteenth and early seventeenth centuries, this chapter suggests that the French disease remained endemic due to Venice's social and sexual networks. Rather than remain isolated within a few neighborhoods along the Rialto or elsewhere, the French disease spread through much of the population because different classes and neighborhoods were connected through intimate relationships. The Venetian elite's practice of social endogamy ironically helped fuel a large number of extra-marital sexual liaisons between noblemen and women of other social classes. Meanwhile, dowry customs, labor migration, women's limited access to paid employment, and widespread sexual violence also contributed to the spread of disease throughout Venice. Much of Venice's highly mobile population experienced changes in sexual partnerships due to migration, death of a partner, or other reasons. Although scholars have often focused on the role of prostitution in the spread of disease, I argue that prostitution alone cannot explain Venice's widespread distribution of disease. As an endemic disease, the French disease was spread through a variety of kinds of sexual relationships, including marriage, concubinage, and relationships between people who called each other "lover" (using the Venetian word *moroso* or the Italian word *amante*). This chapter is therefore a social history of an endemic disease, that is, a study of how social relations produce disease patterns.

Chapter 2 is a study of how the French disease became embedded in Venice's cultural iconography. Historically represented as a beautiful woman, a multivalent symbol of fertility, independence, and vulnerability, the city of Venice faced tremendous military and political risks during the sixteenth century. The symbol of the "beautiful woman," increasingly associated with the threat of sexual disease, invoked Venetian anxiety. I argue that early modern Venetians came to associate the French disease with a beautiful but "promiscuous" woman on the one hand and "dissolute, undisciplined" man (especially a soldier) on the other hand; these associations incorporated Venetian anxieties about their own military vulnerability. This chapter provides an interdisciplinary analysis of how military manuals, medical treatises, art, and literature contributed to the association between beautiful women, danger, undisciplined men, and disease. Perceptions of the French disease thereby became embedded in Venice's cultural constructions of both masculinity and femininity, although feminine representations of the French disease predominated. The image of a beautiful, promiscuous woman galvanized public attention and inspired charitable donations to institutions designed to protect beautiful young girls from seduction and subsequent infection with the French disease. By "quarantining beauty" in these walled institutions on the outskirts of Venice, Venetian authorities hoped to prevent the spread of the French disease, as well as to protect the city from the dangers of moral contagion and preclude potential moral contagion. At the same time, dissolute, undisciplined masculinity represented a threat to Venice's and the Italian peninsula's ability to survive as autonomous states, free from foreign domination. In the wake of foreign invasion and occupation, Venetians and Italians worried about their military security and celebrated ancient Rome's military heroes, such as Scipio Africanus, as symbols of moral and sexual discipline.

Chapter 3 explains how the process of incorporating the French disease into medical and popular narratives of disease causation brought about a shift in perspective from collective to individual responsibility for disease outbreaks. This chapter uses Inquisition trials, criminal records, and medical treatises. I argue that the French disease presented certain challenges to the traditional explanations for the spread of disease, which typically emphasized collective responsibility for epidemic outbreaks, especially in the case of bubonic plague.[47] The French disease was different, however, since it never struck as widely as the plague; in addition, the public as well as medical professions usually traced the disease to sexual activity, and hence to individual behavior. The process of incorporating the French disease into medical and popular narratives therefore involved a change in perceptions about collective versus individual responsibility for disease outbreaks. These two explanatory frameworks, collective and individual, overlapped and coexisted. Nonetheless a subtle change emerged by the late sixteenth century. As Louis Qualtiere and William Slights argue, in literature, such as Shakespeare's *Timon of Athens*, epidemic outbreaks were more often linked to individual behavior, rather than collective moral failings.[48] This chapter explains how stigma related to the French disease fell more heavily on some patients than others, as blame was assigned to certain individuals' behavior. Stigma was not simply an issue of individual behavior, however. Stigma was also embedded in wider social relationships of power, as women and those judged as socially "deviant" were more likely to suffer stigma than men, the powerful, and those who obeyed cultural norms.[49]

Chapter 4 explains how the French disease became embedded in Venice's complex network of charitable institutions, especially the Convertite, the Soccorso, the Zitelle, and the Penitenti, the eighteenth century institution designed to improve on the Convertite's flaws. I argue that these institutions helped "normalize" the French disease by incorporating prevention and care efforts into Venice's institutions that reinforced gender norms and disciplined "deviant" or unconventional sexual behavior by women. These institutions represent a mixed legacy. On the one hand, they reaffirmed Venice's sexual double standard by holding females responsible for sexual disease. Some women and girls were held against their will, even if they were themselves victims of sexual assault. On the other hand, they provided places of shelter, security, and education for females in a world of widespread violence and insecurity. As Sherrill Cohen has argued, these female asylums were prototypes for the later development of women's shelters.[50] They were part of a gendered system of care which demanded moral reform of women in an effort to prevent the French disease or rehabilitate former patients judged to be morally deviant.

1
A Network of Lovers: Sexuality and Disease Patterns in Early Modern Venice

> O my dear Candide! You knew Paquette, that pretty lady's maid to our noble Baroness. In her arms I tasted the delights of paradise, and in turn they have led me to these torments of hell by which you now see me devoured. She had the disease, and may have died of it by now. Paquette was made a present of it by a very knowledgeable Franciscan who had traced it back to its source. For he had got it from an old countess, who had contracted it from a captain in the cavalry, who owed it to a marchioness, who had it from a page, who had caught it from a Jesuit, who, during his noviciate, had inherited it in a direct line from one of Christopher Columbus's shipmates.
>
> Voltaire, *Candide*[1]

Voltaire's eighteenth-century satirical reconstruction of the history of syphilis manages to impugn many of his favorite targets of scorn, especially the clergy. In Voltaire's imagination, disease is passed person-to-person in a huge chain of infection, which reveals all the hypocrisy and decadence of European society. Voltaire is renowned for his anticlericalism, evident here in his suggestion that a Jesuit enjoyed homosexual relations with both a page and one of Columbus's shipmates and that a "humble" Franciscan had a liaison with a countess. Class hierarchies are leveled in Voltaire's chain of infection, as the nobility have sexual relations with their servants. Noticeably absent from Voltaire's description are prostitutes, since European sexual mores are, in his reckoning, sufficiently libertine to transmit disease without relying on prostitution. Although Voltaire's work is an Enlightenment satire using well-known literary tropes of the sexually debauched clergy and the promiscuous noblewoman, it is nonetheless a provocative invitation to examine how sexual connections can link different classes and groups. At least in early modern Venice, the French disease became widespread or endemic throughout the population, across class and ethnic divides, precisely because these sexual links between different groups existed. In short, Voltaire was onto something.

The French disease did not beat a retreat along with the invading French and other European armies, but remained and spread throughout the Italian peninsula and accompanied the returning armies to the rest of Europe. Nor did the disease remain confined to a small group or sub-population in early modern Venice, as sometimes happens with sexually transmitted diseases.[2] In this chapter, I examine mortality data to show that by the mid-sixteenth century, the French disease had spread through much of Venice's population, thereby becoming an endemic disease. I examine Venice's pattern of social networks to explain how Venetians of different social classes, neighborhoods, and ethnic groups were linked through patron–client ties, master–servant relations, concubinage or love relationships, prostitution, and shared housing arrangements, among other ties. Rather than primarily affecting one social class or neighborhood, the French disease became an "equal opportunity" disease in Venice, affecting a broad spectrum of inhabitants, because of Venice's dense social networks that linked various sub-populations.

Meanwhile, the Venetian ruling classes perceived the threat of French disease through the lens of their own preoccupations with protecting their class's exclusivity by forbidding marriage outside their ranks. As Chapter 2 will show, the French disease was a symbol of potential social contagion that beautiful, lower-class women might present if nobleman were ensnared by their beauty or by the illicit practice of love magic. This chapter examines the problems that were largely ignored by the government and the Venetian nobility, especially the problems working-class women faced in developing long-term, stable relationships. Dowry customs and chronic economic insecurity made marriage an often-unrealizable dream. In addition to the marriage customs, women's limited employment options made them dependent on male support, often conditioned on access to a sexual relationship. I refer to these relationships as affective because, the people involved did not describe their relationship as primarily commercial, the exchange of sex for money, but as lovers or "domestic partners." In this chapter, I explore the various routes by which sexually transmitted diseases could travel in sixteenth-century Venice, including how migration, sexual violence and sexual tourism played a role in making the disease endemic and widespread. Venice's unique marriage customs as well as its role as a center of migration created extensive sexual networks which linked the different layers of its sharply differentiated social hierarchy; furthermore, these sexual networks, in addition to prostitution, explain how the French disease traveled through Venetian society and became endemic. Venice's network of social relationships sustained the French disease as an endemic disease.

Who suffered from the French disease?

By the mid-sixteenth century, the French disease was both widespread and widely treated in Venice. Venice was not unique, as the disease was widely regarded as endemic throughout the Italian peninsula.[3] Mortality records can provide more specific information about the distribution of the French disease. It is important to recognize the limitations of this source, since early modern doctors relied on external signs on the body in determining the cause of death.[4] Furthermore, as discussed in the introduction, early modern conceptions of disease differed dramatically from modern conceptions.[5] Determining the cause of death was an imprecise art. Although the cause of death was usually determined by a physician, a physician was not always available, so it is even more difficult to understand what criteria were used to establish a death as caused by the French disease in those cases. It is best, therefore, to regard mortality data as simply providing clues about the distribution of disease in a population, rather than as an accurate representation of mortality rates in early modern Venice. Because the disease became associated with shame during the sixteenth century,[6] families may have exerted pressure not to have deaths attributed to the French disease. Again, the data provide clues, not definitive answers. Although the mortality records theoretically cover all parishes, they should not be regarded as complete: undercounting was probably a problem.[7]

I collected mortality records for 24 non-plague years (1582–91, 1606–10, 1619, 1621, 1623–5, 1636–8, 1641), since during plague years the Health Office's capacity to do anything besides identify plague was severely constrained.[8] Deaths attributed to the French disease always remained low, approximately 15 cases per year but the count dropped lower still after the plague of 1630–1 population decline,[9] because the disease was regarded as curable and seldom fatal. In some cases, the French disease was not the only cause of death listed. Fever was far and away the most common additional cause of death, occurring in 29 out of the 325 deaths; the other conditions (seven total) occurred in only one or two deaths, such as catarrh (two cases), old age (one case, a 70-year-old widow), and tightness of the chest (1 case), among other miscellaneous conditions.

It is important to distinguish between mortality and morbidity data. For a disease that is seldom regarded as fatal, mortality data greatly underestimate the morbidity (extent of disease) in a population. Furthermore, mortality data may misrepresent overall morbidity patterns because they include, by definition, only those who died from disease and therefore the atypical cases: these individuals may have suffered from poorer overall health or had less access to nutrition, housing, and other key determinants of good health. Despite the limitations of these mortality data, the data do nonetheless answer certain important questions about disease distribution: whether the disease was limited to certain populations, neighborhoods, social classes, occupations, or more heavily concentrated among men or women.

The gender distribution is perhaps the most striking data, especially compared to data regarding French disease patients in hospitals. The number of men and women whose deaths were attributed to the French disease is about equal: of the 325 deaths, 157 were women (48.3%) and 168 were men (51.7%) (see Chart 1.1). In Rome's Incurables hospital (San Giacomo) during the same period, women always represented less than 20 percent of admissions. In 1569, for example, a total of 1442 males, but only 335 females, entered the hospital.[10] Venice's records from the Incurables hospital do not survive for the sixteenth and seventeenth centuries, but their eighteenth-century records indicate a similar discrepancy between male and female admissions. In 1769, for example, the hospital admitted 248 men and just 87 women; women therefore accounted for about 26 percent of admissions in that year; in 1771, the percentage was about 30 percent, or 76 women out of 249 admissions.[11] Kevin Siena has shown how access to publicly funded care greatly favored male patients in early modern London, primarily because hospital governors were more sympathetic to male patients and agreed to provide charitable funds for their care.[12] However, the mortality data suggest that women were as likely as men to die from the French disease in early modern Venice. Similar mortality rates indicate either of two propositions: (1) that approximately equal numbers contracted the illness; or (2) that fewer women contracted the disease but suffered a higher mortality rate than men because women lacked adequate access to shelter, food, bed rest, and medical care. Although it is possible that

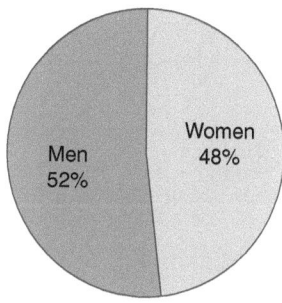

Chart 1.1 Deaths attributed to the French disease by sex

fewer women contracted the disease but more of them died, resulting in these fairly even mortality data, it is much more likely that women and men contracted the disease in roughly even numbers and that women were simply underrepresented in hospitals.

Women who died from the French disease resembled the general population of women in early modern Venice. Of the women whose family status was recorded, the majority of deaths (51.6%) attributed to the French disease were either wives or widows. Wives outnumbered widows, but only slightly: 43 (27.4%) were wives while 38 (24.2%) were widows (see Chart 1.2). The high proportion of married women and widows among the deaths suggests that the French disease was endemic, rather than confined to certain sub-populations. As I discuss later in this chapter, Venice contained a large number of single women, both never married and widowed; in Venice, a woman was as likely to be widowed as married.[13] Women's occupations were recorded only in the case of servants, of whom there were three.

The French disease was regarded as chronic rather than acute, but capable of causing early death, according to the data recorded. Age of death and perceived length of illness varied, but typically patients survived until their late thirties or early forties after a long illness. Two of the deaths attributed to the French disease were infants under one year of age. Except for these two infants, the rest were adult women; the youngest adult woman whose death was attributed to the French disease was 20 years old and the oldest was 73 years old. Most women died in their thirties (approximately 28% of all French disease deaths) or forties (approximately 29% of all French disease deaths; see Table 1.1). Like women infected with the French disease, most men survived into their thirties and forties; 89 (or 53.9%) reached at least the age

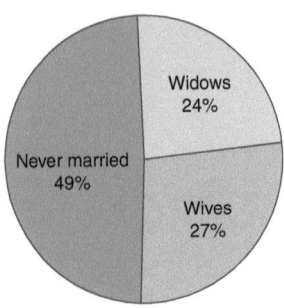

Chart 1.2 Percentage of women by marital status whose deaths were attributed to the French disease

Table 1.1 Women's French disease deaths by age

Age Range for Adult Women	Number of deaths and percentage of total deaths attributed to *mal francese* by age
20–5	18 (11.6%)
26–9	14 (9%)
30–5	28 (18.1%)
36–9	16 (10.3%)
40–9	45 (29%)
50–9	16 (10.3%)
60–9	14 (9%)
70+	4 (2.6%)

Source: Compiled from ASV Provedditori alla Sanità, Busta numbers 814–23, 834–41, 850–4, 867–70 for years 1582–91, 1606–10, 1619, 1621, 1623–5, 1636–8, 1641. Percentages do not add up to 100 due to rounding.

of 36 (see Table 1.2).[14] Both men and women were reported as having endured lengthy illnesses, often of unspecified duration (*"molto tempo"* or *"longamente"*) or several years, typically ranging from 1 to 10 years, with two patients allegedly having had the disease for 20 years.[15] Only a few deaths were reported as the result of a short illness (less than one month), but these were sometimes accompanied by another acute illness, such as fever.[16]

Death records for men indicate that the French disease had infected workers in virtually every sector of the Venetian economy. Fifty-two different occupations or places of work are listed which spanned Venice's social hierarchy, ranging from noblemen (two of them) to merchants (of wine and wool) to highly skilled artisans (such as silk weavers and

Table 1.2 Men's French disease deaths by age

Age Range for Adult Men	Numbers of deaths and percentage of total deaths attributed to mal francese by age
19–25	24 (14.6%)
26–9	16 (9.8%)
30–5	35 (21.3%)
36–9	16 (9.8%)
40–9	48 (29.2%)
50–9	18 (11%)
60–9	5 (3%)
70+	2 (.6%)

Source: Compiled from ASV Provedditori alla Sanità, Busta numbers 814–23, 834–41, 850–4, 867–70 for years 1582–91, 1606–10, 1619, 1621, 1623–5, 1636–8, 1641. Percentages do not add up to 100 due to rounding.

printers) to servants and laborers. Voltaire would not have been surprised to notice that a priest was among those whose death was attributed to the French disease. The list of occupations provides a rich portrait of the diversity of Venice's economy during the period (see Table 1.3), including artisans, merchants, and workers for Venice's various government magistracies, including the *Giustizia vecchia* and the *Avogaria di comune* (workers for government magistracies and incomplete job descriptions, such as a reference only to the shipbuilding factory, the Arsenale, but not the specific occupation, are omitted from Table 1.1). Workers in Venice's cloth industry, both silk and wool, are well represented in this list, as are the range of workers employed at the Arsenale. No fishermen appear on the list, but it is not possible to conclude that this occupation was untouched by the French disease since the sample size is too small to draw such a conclusion.[17]

Mortality data also show that cases of the French disease were spread throughout the city, not just concentrated in one area. Venice was divided into six large administrative districts, called *sestieri*, then subdivided into a total of 70 parishes. Fifty of the city's 70 parishes reported at least one death attributed to the French disease during the years studied. Each of the city's six districts had parishes reporting at least one death due to the French disease (see Table 1.4).

Nonetheless, there were geographical variations in disease distribution. The city's wealthier districts (S. Polo, S. Marco) had fewer parishes reporting at least one death due to the French disease than the city's poorer districts (Cannaregio, Castello). The parishes with the highest number of French disease deaths were densely populated, primarily

24

Table 1.3 Men's French disease deaths by occupation

Occupation	Number of deaths attributed to the French disease
Sailor	5
Galley oarsmen	5
Tailor	4
Silk weaver	4
Silk broker	4
Gondolier	4
Carpenter	4
Wool carder	4
Shoemaker	3
Caulker in the Arsenal	3
Servant	3
Wool worker	3
Dish and pan salesman	4
Cloth weaver	2
Nobleman	2
Barber	2
Mirror-maker	2
Broker	2
Ship-builder at the Arsenal	2
Wine merchant	2
Soldier	2
Printer	1
Shoe repairman	1
Basket-maker	1
Barrel-maker	1
Stonecutter	1
Baker	1
Furrier	1
Priest	1
Mason	1
Porter	1
Master Shipbuilder	1
Tub-maker	1
Bombardier	1
Sword-maker	1
Fruit vendor	1
Prison guard	1
Boot-maker	1
Gold-refiner	1
Soap-maker	1
Wool merchant	1
Used-clothing salesman	1
Cheese-seller	1

Source: Compiled from ASV Provedditori alla Sanità, Busta numbers 814–23, 834–41, 850–4, 867–70 for years 1582–91, 1606–10, 1619, 1621, 1623–5, 1636–8, 1641.

Table 1.4 French disease deaths by neighborhood

Sestiere	Number and % of total parishes per sestiere reporting at least 1 French disease death	Number of total parishes
Cannaregio	10 (83%)	12
Castello	12 (92%)	13
S. Croce	6 (67%)	9
S. Polo	4 (44%)	9
S. Marco	8 (50%)	16
Dorsoduro	10 (91%)	11

Source: Compiled from ASV Provveditori alla Sanità, Busta numbers 814–23, 834–41, 850–4, 867–70 for years 1582–91, 1606–10, 1619, 1621, 1623–5, 1636–8, 1641.

working-class neighborhoods. S. Marcuola had the highest number of French disease deaths (29), followed by S. Martin (22), S. Geremia (17), S. Giovanni in Bragora (17) and S. Moise (14). It is difficult to determine whether that reflects a real difference in distribution of the disease, however. The wealthier districts may have had fewer inhabitants, and therefore the same proportion of disease; or health office officials and parish priests may have been more reluctant to report a death due to the French disease among the city's elite than among the city's poor. Alternatively, the French disease may have been more heavily concentrated among the poor; or the poor may have been more likely to die from the disease, due to inadequate nutrition or lack of access to health care. Although death records do not provide estimates of morbidity or even mortality rates due to the French disease in early modern Venice, they do nonetheless provide a rough portrait. The French disease was evenly distributed between men and women, broadly distributed across the social hierarchy and among a variety of occupations, with perhaps a heavier concentration among the poor, laborers and artisans; and the French disease could be found in the majority of Venetian neighborhoods and parishes.

How did the French disease travel through Venice?

The French disease could travel among many routes that linked the various sub-populations of Venice. After a discussion of source material, interpretation, and social network theory, I trace the major avenues of transmission in three sections: (1) relations among Venice's working classes, laborers, and migrants that linked people of different ethnic groups, occupations, and neighborhoods (as well as linking migrants from rural areas to urban dwellers); (2) relations between the nobility and people of lower classes, including the citizens, a hereditary group immediately below the nobility that often served as government clerks, attorneys, and magistrates; and (3) other factors that influenced sexual behavior and linked different populations, including sexual violence and sexual tourism.

Because of its marriage customs and difficult living and working conditions for the poor, Venice harbored a number of men and women who faced numerous obstacles to marriage but nonetheless found intimate relationships outside of marriage. Court records reveal that these sexual partners often referred to each other as lovers, using either the Italian or Venetian words (*amante, moroso* or *morosa*, respectively).[18] French disease prevention efforts treated these women as prostitutes, thereby ignoring these women's perception of themselves as potential wives and often making it shameful for women to seek treatment. Whether by choice or by necessity, women and men of the popular classes created and inhabited an enormously fluid social world. Venice's working classes and noblemen experienced intimate relationships prior to, sometimes during, and after marriage (during widowhood), thereby providing many avenues for the transmission of the French disease. In addition, sexual violence played a role in the spread of disease, while the city's reputation as a haven of beautiful courtesans attracted sexual tourists.[19] The French disease became endemic partly because the city's economy, social structure and customs, and social dynamics helped foster and sustain disease transmission.

Although this chapter primarily focuses on heterosexual routes of transmission, homosexual relations provided another route for disease to travel through Venetian society. Although same-sex sexual relations were not officially permissible in Venice, the Venetian government relaxed its enforcement of the anti-sodomy laws during the late sixteenth and early seventeenth centuries compared to its more vigorous prosecution in the fourteenth and fifteenth centuries. "Active partners" were burned alive until 1446, while later they were decapitated and then burned. "Passive partners" in Venice endured lighter penalties, such as fines, or might go free. This heavy state policing of sexuality helped create what Guido Ruggiero has called an "illicit culture of sexuality" in fifteenth-century Venice, in which illegal sexual relations such as rape, sodomy, and fornication nonetheless flourished.[20] Sodomy most often referred to anal sex between men, but was a term that could also refer to anal or oral sex between men or between men and women.[21] Anxious about fertility, especially after the decimations of the Italian Wars, Italian Renaissance writers and government officials worried about anal sex even if it occurred between a man and a woman since it did not produce children.[22]

As in Florence, sexual relationships between men in Venice were relatively common during adolescence and early adulthood, the period of life before men married.[23] Typically, an unmarried man in his late twenties or early thirties might enjoy a sexual relationship with an adolescent male aged 15–18. The younger male assumed the "passive" or receptive role in the relationship, which was regarded as feminine and therefore not suitable for an adult male in full possession of his masculinity. Men in these relationships did not have a "homosexual identity," that is, they did not define themselves in terms of their sexual desires for men nor confine their sexual interests to males.[24] In addition to the age difference, there might be a class difference between the lovers as well. Men involved in homosexual relationships might also be involved in heterosexual relations as well, sometimes at the same time or later in marriage. Although homosexual relationships were supposed to occur only prior to marriage, in practice these relations might continue throughout a man's life. For example, Venice's Council of Ten complained in 1516 that men in their forties, fifties, and even sixties were paying other men to penetrate them, thereby assuming the passive role which was supposed to be reserved for younger men only.[25] Homosexual relations between men of different age groups and social classes provided another means through which disease could travel through Venetian society. Furthermore, because it was unusual to engage exclusively in homosexual relations in early modern Venice, homosexual and heterosexual networks were overlapping, rather than mutually exclusive, thereby providing greater opportunities for disease to spread through the population.

Historical Sources and Interpretation

Information about intimate relationships usually is available in historical records where they appeared when these relationships dissolved and conflict erupted, with one or both parties appearing in court. For example, a relationship between a nobleman and a working-class woman could have several possible outcomes, each leaving a different kind of historical record: the nobleman could have paid for her entry into one of the female asylums, such as the Convertite or Casa del Soccorso, a situation that will be described in Chapter 4;[26] he could provide a marriage dowry for her to marry another man;[27] he could abandon her with no resources; and, finally and rarely, he himself could marry her.[28] Each of these possible endings will be discussed below, after explaining the methodological significance of these records. For this chapter, I have used the trial records of the Holy Office from 1570 to 1650 (cases from 1593 to 1610 are missing from the archive), the sentences from the *Esecutori contra la Bestemmia*, and the records from the Health Office (the *Sanità*). In addition, historians such as Joanne Ferraro, Alexander Cowan, Guido Ruggiero, and Gabriele Martini have found evidence of intimate relationships outside of marriage from their work in the Patriarchal Archives and the records of the Holy Office.[29] That traces of these relationships exist in the records of several bureaucratic offices, state and ecclesiastical, and in different contexts provides strong evidence that intimate relationships outside of marriage were not uncommon. What these sources do not provide, however, is a reliable measure of how common these relationships were: we can make no guesses about the numbers of men and women involved. Criminal records and Inquisition trials also provide insight into the cultural conflicts and anxieties of early modern Venetians by showing how these women and men explained their relationship to different authorities.[30] In addition to trial records and petitions to state and ecclesiastical courts, parish census records and laws provide an indication of the social context in which Venetians formed relationships.

Relationships outside of marriage have often been mistakenly described as prostitution based on the use of the word *meretrice*, a term which includes but is not limited to prostitution. In fact, the word *meretrice* was a moral category that referred to a woman's sexual activities outside of marriage rather than an occupation or commercial transaction. In 1543, the Venetian Senate defined the word *meretrici* as those women who "not being married have commerce, and practice with one, or more men" (commerce or *commercio* being used in the sense of intercourse, as in "carnal commerce"). *Meretrici* were also defined as "those who being married do not live with their husbands but stay separately, and have commerce with one or more men."[31] Hence any woman who had sex outside of marriage, whether in a long-term relationship with one man, or an adulterous relationship, was called a *meretrice*. Lucia Ferrante found that in Bologna, the majority of women named as *meretrici* in city registers were the exclusive concubines of one man, rather than street walkers who had multiple sexual partners. These concubines' relationships often endured for years.[32] Similarly, in seventeenth-century London, communities exercised considerable control over sexuality in order to prevent God's wrath against morality. Reputation and "common fame" in the neighborhood weighed more heavily than legalistic definitions of prostitution as a venture in which sex was exchanged for money; sexual misconduct was the principal concern, which included adultery and even aiding and abetting the immorality of others.[33] It is therefore important not to assume that every woman named as a *meretrice* in early modern records was a prostitute in the sense of having multiple paying male clients. Mistakenly referring to all of these women as prostitutes leads to an exaggeration of the numbers of women involved in prostitution and its role in the transmission of disease.

My contribution to the lively scholarship on sexuality and intimate relationships in early modern Venice is to argue that Venice developed a pattern of sexual relationships or sexual networks that linked different sub-populations and facilitated the transmission of disease, thereby shifting attention from prostitution alone. Contemporary social theory about social networks and the transmission of disease sheds light on Venice's situation. Once an initial "core group," such as soldiers or prostitutes, becomes infected, social network theory explains whether a sexually transmitted disease will move relatively slowly and infect small numbers of people, or spread quickly and permeate a society. Societies that are divided into distinctive and isolated sub-populations, such as those with deep ethnic or religious divides, are less likely to provide the conditions for the rapid spread of sexually transmitted diseases through the entire society; whereas societies that have highly dense social networks, where individuals maintain large social networks that link various sub-populations, are better conduits for the transmission of these diseases.[34] "Density" is a term that refers to the number of links between individuals in a given society. A society with highly dense social networks is one in which individuals maintain a large number of social ties.[35]

Social network theory developed largely within the field of sociology, partly by scholars trying to understand the nature of epidemic disease.[36] Prior to the development of social network theory, its practitioners argue, epidemiologists understood populations as "amorphous agglomerations of randomly interacting individuals." That approach, despite its theoretical simplicity, was sufficient for understanding an epidemic disease spread through casual, fleeting contact, such as with influenza and malaria.[37] Sexually transmitted diseases presented challenges, since they are not transmitted randomly. Instead, disease transmission requires intimate, and even repeated, personal contact, therefore requiring a more nuanced understanding of populations.[38] Because relationships are the key unit of investigation, social network analysis begins by studying the relationships between people, rather than by examining attributes such as class, ethnicity, gender, and neighborhood of origin.[39]

Social network theory helps explain why sexually transmitted diseases, such as HIV/AIDS, remain relatively confined to certain neighborhoods and sub-populations or spread more widely. For example, among migrants to the UK, HIV/AIDS seldom moves beyond a particular neighborhood, since people usually choose sexual partners of the same nationality, background and even neighborhood as themselves, hence there are relatively few links or "bridges" between various ethnicities to spread disease. In the UK, people of the same nationality typically live in the same neighborhood.[40] By contrast, migrants to the Netherlands do not live in neighborhoods segregated by nationality; sexual relationships between members of different ethnic groups are more common, thereby providing a link between different populations for the diffusion of disease.[41] Early modern Venice more closely resembles the contemporary Netherlands than the UK in having links between different ethnic groups and sub-populations.

Social and economic issues, such as labor migration, also affect the transmission of disease. Poor treatment of migrant workers can have devastating effects on the transmission of disease, especially in the case of HIV/AIDS in southern Africa. Subject to strict rules under the apartheid regime, miners in South Africa were not allowed to bring their families to the towns where they lived 11 months of the year. Men from Botswana, Zaire, and throughout southern Africa lived in crowded hostels with few opportunities for recreation, aside from drinking in local bars and visiting prostitutes.[42] The result is that migrant men were much more likely than non-migrants to become infected with HIV (25.9% of migrant vs. 12.7% of non-migrant men).[43] Wives remaining at home were also more likely to become infected with HIV than the wives of non-migrant men. These wives were not necessarily exposed by their husbands, but also by other partnerships that sometimes developed during their husbands' absence.[44] The conditions under which this labor migration occurred exposed miners and their families to HIV and are among key factors behind the explosive growth of HIV infection in southern Africa, where HIV/AIDS prevalence is highest in the world. On a smaller scale and with less restrictive laws, Venice was also a major center for seasonal and permanent migration, the conditions of which contributed at least partially to disease transmission.

Unfortunately, the data from early modern Italy do not provide a complete picture of any individual's entire social network. This chapter therefore draws insights from, rather than rigorously applying, social network analysis. Based on case studies from archival records and a highly developed historiography of Renaissance Italian social relations, the evidence suggests that early modern Italy was a society of relatively dense social networks for several reasons: the ubiquity of patron–client ties,[45] of master–servant relations, [46] and, in urban areas, the prevalence of renting bedroom space or bed-space, all of which provided links between Italians of different classes, ethnicities, neighbors and even cities of residence.[47] At the same time, however, Venice had its share of social divisions: in particular, the isolation of the Jewish population in the ghetto, as well as neighborhoods dominated by a particular occupation, notably the fishermen known as the *Nicolotti* who lived in the parishes of San Niccolò and San Angelo Raffaele.[48] In addition, noblewomen's social networks and geographical mobility were circumscribed, especially in Venice, where they were seldom allowed to leave the house and were carefully supervised.[49] Aside from these important exceptions, however, sexual relationships in Venice developed within the widespread social networks that linked different social class, ethnicities, neighborhoods and even cities.

Intimacy among the working classes

Impermanence: Mobility and early death

As a center of trade and industry, Venice attracted skilled and unskilled workers, female and male, from its territories on the mainland as well as from other city-states, with large numbers from the Veneto, Friuli, Lombardy, and the Istrian coast. Women were more likely to make Venice their permanent home, whereas men, if they were skilled artisans, often moved from city to city in pursuit of higher salaries.[50] Both males and females were usually unmarried and migrated by themselves to Venice. During the mid- to late sixteenth century, in Venice's thriving silk industry, for example, artisans could easily move several times during their lives.[51] Although it is difficult to find definitive evidence that geographic mobility increased the likelihood of Venetians' practicing "serial monogamy," a series of successive relationships, or perhaps even overlapping relationships with sexual partners in different cities, it is one possible explanation for the references to artisan and working-class lovers who never married.[52] Early death also meant that Venetians could expect to have more than one sexual partner during their lives, even if they had married. For example, a certain Cecilia who lived on the Giudecca lost her "*moroso*" (lover) named Bernardo during the plague of 1630–1, then married a gondolier who also died, leaving her a widow in her thirties.[53] Multiple successive relationships, with the possibility of overlapping relationships in the case of migrants, greatly increase the chances that sexually transmitted diseases will spread widely through a population.[54]

Long-term sexual relationships outside of marriage were fairly common among Venice's working classes. It is striking how often Venetians used the word *moroso* or *morosa*, even when the woman has been denounced as a *meretrice* to the Holy Office of the Inquisition. The denunciation against Francesca from Bari, for example, mentioned her practice of love magic and referred to her as a *"meretrice,"* but her sister described her steady relationship with a man named Camillo, her *"moroso."*[55] Felicita, a Greek woman living in Murano, is referred to as a *meretrice* because she is not married, or according to one witness, "she is not married to my knowledge, if she were not married outside of Murano, but in Murano she is not married; she has a certain fellow who keeps her called Giulio dal Tesdesco."[56] In this case, the speaker's use of the word *meretrice* seems to hinge on the fact that she is not married, or at least not locally recognized as married, and has a sexual relationship with one clearly identified man who pays at least some of her expenses. This relationship, like others in court records, more closely resembles concubinage than prostitution.

Sometimes the female partner nursed expectations of marriage that were never realized.[57] In the words of Marina Facchinetti in reference to a certain Francesco Nocenti, "Yes, I know him. This man was my lover (*moroso*). It's this man who was married last August, even though he had promised to take me for his wife."[58] As she explained during her trial, it was her desperation over Francesco's abandonment of her that drove her to turn to magical practices to determine her future: to marry someone else, go to the temporary shelter the Casa del Soccorso or enclose herself at the Convertite.[59] Denounced as *meretrici*, trial records often indicate that these many of these women had only one lover at a time and often hoped to marry their lover. The male partner, however, may have enjoyed more than one sexual partnership at a time, as this example indicates. His concurrent relationships increased the chances of spreading disease, if he or either of his sexual partners were exposed.[60]

Venice's demographic composition made it difficult, if not impossible, for some women to find marriage partners, not sexual partners. The number of single women in Venice exceeded that of single men; interestingly, of these single people, twice as many women headed households as men. Based on Monica Chojnacka's work on household censuses (*status animarum*), at least 8672 single adult women (never married) and 4924 widows (not remarried) lived in the parishes that were counted during the census (only two-thirds of the parishes were counted), out of a total population of 94,862 persons (men, women, and children). Approximately 14 percent of Venice's population represented unmarried or widowed adult women. Given that parish censuses tended to underestimate the numbers of poor residents and recent immigrants, it seems likely that these parishes harbored even more single women than the records indicate.[61]

Working-class Venetians could meet each other and develop relationships in a variety of ways. Immigrants to the city often rented a spare room in an apartment and interacted closely with their landlord or landlady and other tenants. Boarding houses also existed, but they were less common than a more informal arrangement. Venetian officials feared that sexual relationships might develop between a landlady and male tenants and tried to prevent women from running boarding houses, but in practice it was difficult, in fact impossible, to prohibit Venetian women from renting single rooms to male boarders.[62] For example, in spring 1642,[63] 30 out of 288 (10.4%) artisan households in the working-class parish of S. Giovanni in Bragora had a temporary tenant resident in their household. Temporary female tenants were not officially recorded, although anecdotal evidence from trial records suggests that women also took up temporary residence within a household. "Foreigners" were also a significant presence in artisan households in S. Giovanni in Bragora, with 57 out of 288 (19.8%) artisan households reporting the presence of a foreigner.[64]

Venice was a vibrant city, filled with markets and celebration of frequent festivals, thereby providing multiple opportunities for newcomers to meet and form relationships. Female networks provided one opportunity for women to build alliances for support in time of need,[65] while relationships with men of equal or higher social standing provided another opportunity. These links between newly arrived migrants and residents, as well between the working classes, enabled the French disease to travel from one ethnic group to another and from one neighborhood to another.

Sexual intimacy across the class divide

Liaisons between noblemen and non-nobles

The French disease could also travel across social classes, even in a city as rigidly hierarchical as Venice. Ironically, the Venetian nobility's preoccupation with social exclusion may have inadvertently helped fuel the spread of the French disease. Politically, Venice was a closed society that took great efforts to preserve the political privileges of the few. Part of the Venetian patriciate's strategy to maintain power for the few was to restrict ways of acquiring noble status through marriage and reproduction. The political mythology of a "pure" ruling class was literally enacted by informally adopting endogamous practices in the fourteenth century, then by making endogamy part of the constitutional principles of government in a series of laws passed during the fifteenth and sixteenth centuries. Marriage between a nobleman and non-noblewoman, if the union produced children, resulted in non-noble children. In order to avoid this situation, the Venetian nobility practiced the highest known rate of endogamy in early modern Europe.[66] Law and custom combined to keep most young noblemen from marrying and from marrying outside their class. Nothing, however, prevented them from finding female companionship outside of marriage. Political exclusiveness ironically brought about fluid social conditions and the development of cross-class social and sexual networks, providing another route for the French disease to travel.

Young Venetian noblemen found themselves in a difficult predicament if they sought sexual relations only within marriage. Many noblemen faced years or even decades of bachelorhood. Among nobles, only one son per generation was allowed to marry. This practice limited the pool of legitimate children who could inherit wealth.[67] Venice's marriage practices also inadvertently increased the pool of unmarried young noblemen, whose options for sexual relationships were often limited to women they could not marry, unless they were willing to forfeit their children's status as nobility. Meanwhile, as many as one-third to one-half of all of Venice's noblewomen were shut up in convents, which provided inexpensive alternatives to marriage dowries for the daughters of noble families keen on preserving wealth and social status.[68] These women were therefore not available for social or sexual relationships, especially after the Council of Trent imposed strict cloister on all convents (see Chapter 4). As scholars have already shown, Venetian noblemen resolved their predicament by developing sexual relationships with women (or men) from the lower classes.[69]

Although relatively few in number, noblemen maintained wide social networks as both patrons and clients with all levels of Venice's social hierarchy. Between 1500 and 1575, the number of noblemen ranged between 2500 and 3000.[70] They alone had the privilege of sitting on Venice's Great Council, in which magistrates were elected, as well as the privilege of obtaining membership to other councils. The Great Council officially closed its ranks in 1297, making it practically impossible, except in extraordinary cases, to become a member of the nobility. As a result, the Venetian patriciate became a closed, hereditary caste.[71] The primary power of the noblemen was political: access to office-holding, the ability to grant favors, the ability to vote and influence policy, and centrality within patron–client networks constituted the major sources of power.

Differences in wealth among noblemen were often substantial. To be noble did not necessarily mean to be rich, nor even to be comfortable. But it did mean not sinking to the level of absolute poverty, homelessness, and degradation that was the lot of Venice's unskilled laborers when they fell on hard times. Because of the importance of maintaining their status as the ruling elite, the wealthier members of the nobility had an incentive to keep their poorer brethren from resembling vagabonds. Charity was given to the nobility before all others, a practice that the future Cardinal Gasparo Contarini defended in 1516 as a pious act, since poverty was not the nobility's natural condition and, because of it, they suffered even more greatly than others.[72] The nobility's protection from extreme poverty was one manifestation of a broader political process and mythology—the idea that only the Republic of Venice, with its pure and immaculate ruling class, would enjoy permanent political stability, free of the factional strife that plagued other Italian cities.[73]

For a laundress or bead stringer, recently emigrated from the countryside, for example, the social gap between herself and the poorest nobleman was typically visible and wide. A liaison with a nobleman was a source of considerable fantasy for many women of the popular classes and of anxiety for noble families, who feared social contamination through intermarriage with their social inferiors. The anxieties produced by these relationships partially fuelled both the practice and repression of "love magic," a means of seduction or of securing the affections and loyalty of another. Seldom did liaisons between noblemen and working-class women end in marriage, but neither were these relationships simple exchanges of sex for money, or prostitution, a word that obscures the meaning of these relationships to both parties. Noblemen provided access to the use of their name, a network of alliances, a permanent place in one of the city's asylums for women, or financial support. In addition to sex, women provided long-term companionship and domestic services. These relationships had cultural significance beyond the immediate participants in providing the context for the growth of love magic prosecutions and the development of a new literary genre, the fairy tale known as "rise tale" in which a commoner gains access to wealth through marriage.[74]

A relationship with a non-noble woman could provide access to sexual and affective relationships that were formally denied to some noblemen. As proof of this, married noblemen sometimes kept concubines, a practice with a long history on the Italian peninsula.[75] Concubines were tolerated in law and practice as a kind of inferior or parallel marriage. As Emlyn Eisenach argues, a nobleman communicated his wealth, status and power by keeping a concubine: only the wealthy could afford the expense, and the concubine, unlike his socially equal wife, was completely at his disposal.[76]

Wives who found their husbands' concubines or mistresses intolerable could accuse their husbands of having infected them with the French disease and seek a marital separation. A physician's testimony that the wife in question had indeed contracted the French disease was necessary and provided solid, physical evidence in the eyes of the court that some marital abuse had occurred.[77] Chapter 3 provides a more detailed discussion of the fears that Venetian women had about the possibility of being infected by their adulterous husbands.[78] Again, it is difficult to estimate how widespread adulterous relations were, and impossible to know how many of them actually resulted in disease transmission. All we can say with confidence is that it was another route for disease to travel.

Meanwhile, lower-class women ironically found themselves in a situation similar to that of noblemen, since marriage customs restricted their access to suitable marriage partners. By 1400, the dowry system had become so entrenched that Renaissance Italians could scarcely imagine marriage without it.[79] The dowry system linked the exchange of goods and money to marriage and sexuality. Although dowry was intended to provide financial support for marriage and economic security for widows, it could easily become the reason for marriage. By the sixteenth century, prospective husbands overlooked the past sexual histories of potential brides if they brought sizeable dowries. Occasionally, as discussed below, women acquired a marriage dowry through a sexual relationship with another man. The dowry system inadvertently placed the financial burden of marriage formation on females.[80] Theoretically, of course, it was the fathers of prospective brides who were supposed to supply the dowry, which would then be given to the groom upon marriage. In practice, however, women of the working classes—especially Venice's sizeable population of immigrants from Venice's mainland territories, Greece, and other Italian states—came from families who could not afford to provide a dowry for them at all and therefore had to earn it themselves.[81] Women therefore had to earn their own dowries in an economy that restricted their access to many types of employment.[82] The dowry system thereby inadvertently enhanced tensions it was supposed to resolve: instead of relieving financial pressures, it simply moved them from the young couple to the single woman and her family.[83]

Although I have primarily emphasized the barriers that noblemen and working-class women faced if they wanted to marry, it did occasionally happen. The practice of "secret marriage" became a viable option during the seventeenth century, although its very existence underscores the social pressure these couples faced from their families not to marry. For noble families eager to maintain their assets and exclusivity, lovers were more acceptable than wives from lower classes. For example, in 1581, when Marco Dandolo, the scion of a wealthy noble family, married the courtesan Andriana Savorgnan, his family lost little time in accusing her of practicing love magic to win their son's affections. As Guido Ruggiero explains, Dandolo's family and friends asserted that he had "lost his ability to act independently and was completely at the mercy of Andriana."[84] Belief in the extraordinary power of beautiful women and of love magic made Venice's ruling classes fearful of women farther down the social hierarchy.[85]

Technically legal, secret marriages circumvented potential family opposition by not being celebrated in the bride's home parish, nor publicly announced previously through publication of the banns, nor recorded in the parish register. Instead, a priest performed the public ceremony before witnesses, thereby fulfilling the church's requirements for a legal marriage, and the marriage was registered in a book of secret marriages.[86] The sons of these unions did not become members of the nobility, but the daughters could marry a nobleman.[87]

Typically, the marriages followed a long period of mutual acquaintance, more than a decade, the longest having been 36 years. Some women were the concubines of a nobleman, others simply had their expenses paid in a separate residence, a few had been employed as domestic servants when the relationship began, some were described as a "friend," and at least one was called a *meretrice* by angry members of the nobleman's family.[88] Between 1633 and 1699, records exist for 330 cases of secret marriage, many of them between non-nobles, who had their own reasons for keeping marriages secret. For example, widows were eager to protect their access to their late husbands' houses, which they risked losing if they remarried.[89] The fantasy of marrying a nobleman was seldom realized, but reality did not necessarily diminish hope and may have even encouraged women to form sexual liaisons outside of marriage.[90] These cases provide further evidence of sexual relationships that drew Venetians of different classes together into a larger sexual network. In addition, as mentioned before, sexual links between classes included homosexual as well as heterosexual relations.

Widening the social network: Subsequent marriage to another

A nobleman's lover sometimes had another possibility besides marriage to the nobleman himself: he might provide a dowry for her to marry a different man, thereby inadvertently widening Venice's sexual network. For example, the nobleman Andrea Dolfin not only provided a marriage dowry for his former lover, Laura Belfante, but also actually arranged the marriage himself. After giving birth to his child, and being eight months' pregnant with his second child, Laura Belfante found herself in a forced marriage to a farm-worker. Only two weeks later, she hired a lawyer and filed for an annulment, but was unsuccessful.[91] Noblemen sometimes tried to end their relationships with women by foisting them off on working-class men, who apparently readily married them for their dowry. Occasionally women were able to contest these marriages successfully. As Joanne Ferraro explains, some women preferred to be the lovers of noblemen rather than the wives of their social equals: hopes of upward social mobility led them to reject marriages to peers.[92] Other women accepted this resolution to their relationship and willingly entered a marriage with a low-status male, who was content with the dowry the match brought even if his new bride had been another man's lover.[93] A sexually transmitted disease could thereby theoretically travel from nobleman to working-class lover to her future working-class husband.

A woman who did not accept marriage to a working-class man could potentially find herself abandoned with no support, but the results might have been the same in terms of potential for disease transmission since she was still available for new relationships. In 1667, for example, 43-year-old Zanetta Molina was struggling to make ends meet after her most recent lover, a gondolier, had abandoned her. Her last name, Molina, she received not from her father or from a husband (apparently she never married). As she explained to the Holy Office where she was standing trial on accusations of practicing sorcery, she received her name "good and true" from a nobleman of the Molin family who had taken her virginity years earlier.[94] Given Molina's age, it may have been decades since she lost her virginity. Her continued insistence on affiliating herself with this noble name in the face of inquisitors from the Holy Office suggests that the name itself had some meaning. His name was doing her little good in practical terms: she was unable to retain the affections of the gondolier, even after she prepared a meal of red rice (*risi rossi*), made with her own menstrual blood, in a vain attempt to bind his love to her.[95] The serial relationships, right across Venice's hierarchy from nobleman to gondolier, show how Venice's society provided an easy path for disease to travel.

The married concubine

A nobleman could also introduce his lover and her kin to an entirely different social network, thereby expanding her and her family's opportunities for both material and social advancement. The case of Isabella Novaglia provides an interesting example. While on trial in 1640 before the Holy Office for practicing various forms of magic, Novaglia forthrightly explained her history of sexual liaisons outside of marriage, which began with her husband arranging her first tryst when the couple's assets were finished. "While I was married to my husband I was good, and well-off for five continuous years. But because in this time he had squandered everything of mine, he himself gave me in hand to a gentleman, who was from the house of Querini. In this time, and afterwards [the gentleman Querini] always helped me. Afterwards I attached myself to a merchant, who is Signor Pietro Raspi of the Merceria. And then I did according to what occasion required. And after Raspi I attached myself to said old man [Francesco Michelion, orderly at customs, who was previously mentioned in the trial], and with others according to what opportunity threw open to me."[96] Novaglia's testimony stands out for a couple of reasons: first, she was married; second, she describes a descent into what appears to have been prostitution, with her husband acting as pimp. Even so, the relationship with the nobleman Querini was more complex and enduring than the term prostitution suggests. In fact, the offer of friendship after the sexual relationship is suggestive of another kind of relationship, a patron–client relationship.

Other witnesses confirmed Isabella's version of the story and supplied more details suggestive of a patron–client bond between Isabella's husband and Querini. Giovanni Battiramo, a 30-year-old solicitor, testified that he had met Isabella and her husband three years before, through an introduction by Zorzi Querini. By that time, Isabella and Querini were no longer lovers. Querini introduced Battiramo to Isabella's husband so that they could do business using Isabella's dowry.[97] Neither Battiramo nor Isabella described their relationship as sexual. Instead, it was a business relationship between himself and her husband, with Isabella's newly reconstituted dowry providing the capital. Patron–client ties have long been recognized as fundamental to the organization of Renaissance Italian city-states, so enduring that they have been called "deep structures."[98] Although some scholars have argued that patron–client ties operated chiefly among the political elite,[99] others have emphasized how widespread patronage was, extending well beyond the political classes to link artisans and workers in an informal chain toward the centers of political power.[100] Even if a nobleman could not provide financial resources himself, he could introduce his clients to others who could. Patrons sometimes received bribes from potential clients, a powerful motive for a patron to attract more clients.[101] All three parties, or at least Querini and Isabella's husband, apparently benefited from the arrangement. Querini enjoyed sexual relations and expanded his network of loyal clients, while Isabella's husband had access to a new business opportunity and the potential to earn more money. Her dowry thereby became a kind of renewable resource, once squandered it could be reconstituted through her sexual services.

This practice of offering one's wife as a sexual partner to a well-connected patron was not isolated or confined to Venice.[102] In Verona, two women sought separations from their husbands after their husbands urged them to become the concubines of wealthy merchants or gentlemen in order to earn more money.[103] In another similar case in Venice, Madalena, a gondolier's wife, fled her husband, who had arranged meetings alone in his boat with a certain spice merchant in exchange for money. This case demonstrates the limits of socially acceptable sexual behavior in early modern Venice, since the gondolier received widespread criticism from neighbors who came to testify on his wife's behalf.[104] Working-class men may occasionally have arranged for their wives to become the lovers of wealthier men in exchange for money, but this behavior seems to have been exceptional and not widely tolerated. Concubinage was socially acceptable only as long as the female partner was unmarried, but a few people nonetheless transgressed social norms.

Abuse of the master–servant relationship

Another cross-class relationship that could occasionally foster the development of sexual relations was the master–servant tie. It is difficult to overstate the importance of master–servant relations in early modern Europe: as Dennis Romano argues, "the master–servant tie was one of the fundamental relationships that characterized European society before the era of the French Revolution."[105] Households of varying wealth and status kept servants, from that of humble artisans and of stigmatized prostitutes to that of the wealthiest noble families and, of course, the doge himself.[106] Nonetheless, the relationship between master and servant involved power and influence: when the masters were artisans, their servants came from more humble backgrounds.

The Venetian government was concerned about the potential for sexual relations to develop between masters and servants, thereby threatening the honor of the ruling classes. Household treatises frequently made comparisons between the governance of the household and the governance of the state: the household was not the "private," domestic realm, separate and distinct from government, but rather it was government on a smaller, more immediate, scale. Sexual activity threatened to disrupt households and therefore, literally and metaphorically, the state itself. Wives could become jealous and angry if their husbands engaged in sexual relations with servants, whereas unmarried men who slept with servants threatened the hierarchical relationships within the household (and the city at large) by allowing servants to become a kind of surrogate spouse. Despite explicit penalties against master–servant sexual relations, abuses did occur.[107] Women of the popular classes were at a clear disadvantage in laying charges of sexual abuse against the nobility. Even clear-cut cases of violent rape with abductions were scarcely regarded as crimes if the rapes were committed by noblemen against lower-class women.[108] Nonetheless, evidence does exist that sexual relationships developed.

Evidence about sexual relations between masters and servants more often comes from various criminal records. Gasparo de Medici, a man approximately 40 years old, appeared before the Holy Office of the Inquisition on several charges, including allegations that he had had sexual relations with Maria, his female servant, beginning when she was about nine or ten years old and continuing for a decade. He did not deny that the two had sexual relations (Maria had given birth to his child). He defended himself by saying that he did not want to go to confession during this time, since the confessor would tell him that he was in mortal sin for having a concubine: not wanting to abandon her and disobey his confessor, he decided not to go to confession at all.[109] Defloration cases also provide evidence of sexual relations between masters and servants. In March 1627, for example, the domestic servant

Emilia (last name not provided) brought charges against her employer, Bortholomio Agazi, a spice merchant, for having taken her virginity on the promise that he would provide her with a dowry, which he then failed to do.[110] These sexual relationships cannot be understood simply as "commercial sex," since a prostitute could not have won this kind of case. The crime of taking a woman's virginity could only be successfully prosecuted if the woman had a well-established reputation in the neighborhood as a virgin and honorable woman. Although it is difficult to know the frequency with which sexual relationships developed, domestic-servant relations were nonetheless one more route through which disease could travel across Venetian society.

Sexual violence and sexual tourism

Of course, not all sexual relations in Venice were consensual. Based on criminal records, sexual violence was widespread in early modern Venice and provided yet another conduit for disease.[111] During the eighteenth century, the French disease was used as evidence of rape in court cases in which young girls were the victims of crimes; I discuss these cases in Chapter 4 in the context of new institutions to prevent and control the French disease.

During the sixteenth and seventeenth centuries, rapes were committed by men of every social rank against women of every social rank. Noblemen, however, were seldom prosecuted for their crimes.[112] Gang rape was one of the ways in which young men in late medieval and early modern Europe could acquire "the privilege of masculinity" and be admitted to the ranks of adult men.[113] Prosecution of rapists varied according to the age, status, and reputation of the victim. Rapists of children were given harsh sentences; rapists of widows less so, while the rape of a single, working-class woman of marriageable age "could virtually disappear as a crime."[114] The impact of sexual violence is discussed again in Chapter 4, which describes how female asylums provided shelter from a violent society where vulnerable women, especially widows and orphan girls, were targets for rape and humiliation. Although it is difficult to estimate with precision the extent of sexual violence in early modern Venice, court records surely underestimate the crime, given the combination of shame, humiliation, and the enormous burden of proof placed on the victims.

Rape accounts for only part of the sexual cases involving young girls. Economic coercion was certainly a factor, as well as parental pressure if the family had limited resources. It is difficult to say whether Venice's young girls were particularly at risk of sexual defilement and potential infection with the French disease on account of a widespread rumor that sexual intercourse with a virgin could cure an infected male.[115] The motives of men who had sexual relations with young girls were not discussed. Saint Disdier reported in 1635 that foreign men arrived in Venice to buy sexual favors from young virgin girls: it is not clear whether they were trying to cure themselves of the French disease, or simply protect themselves from contracting it by having sexual relations with a virgin. According to Disdier, the going price for a young girl's virginity was 100 or 200 ducats, sufficient to provide a marriage dowry. Men arrived in Venice specifically for the purpose of finding these girls: one man complained that he was shown a girl so thin and young that her breasts were not yet developed.[116] Male demand for sexual services, as well as Venice's reputation as a haven of female beauty, was decisive in fuelling Venice's commercial sex industry.

By the eighteenth century, however, desire to avoid contracting the French disease definitely motivated men to have sex with young girls. For example, the writer Jean-Jacques Rousseau (1712–78) spent time in Venice during the 1740s and wrote about his fears of contracting the French disease. He and a friend came up with a plan to spare themselves the consequences of disease by "investing" in a prepubescent virgin female, paying for part of her education, and waiting for her to achieve sexual maturity so they could take their pleasure with her. Although Rousseau himself found that his paternal feelings for the girl ultimately interfered with his ability to consummate this relationship, others, most notably the notorious writer and libertine, Giacomo Casanova (1725–98), were not so circumspect. One young girl's mother allegedly sold her virginity to Casanova; when the girl refused to have sex, he beat her up. It was not until the 1780s that Venetian authorities began to recognize the impact of these sexual relationships on the child's sensibilities, rather than focusing more narrowly on the loss of virginity and subsequent marriage prospects for the girl.[117]

This chapter has traced the routes by which the French disease could travel through Venetian society, showing the sexual links between Venice's different neighborhoods, ethnic groups, and social classes. Venice was a welcoming city for the French disease: despite considerable discussion about the exclusivity of the Venetian elite, or about the myriad ethnic divisions and diverse neighborhoods, in practice the city provided ample opportunity for the disease to disperse to all of its neighborhoods, rich and poor, in male and female bodies that spoke Venetian dialect, Florentine Italian, Greek, German, and many other tongues. The economic, cultural, and social context, including elite marriage practices, dowry, and labor migration, all conspired to make long-term sexually exclusive unions difficult to maintain in practice, and all but unattainable for certain groups, such as young, poor women recently migrated from the countryside. Noblemen and wealthy men did not always demonstrate a proclivity for long-term sexually exclusive unions, since keeping a concubine brought status and prestige. Venetians enjoyed or at least consented to a variety of sexual practices, oral and anal, in both homosexual and heterosexual relationships. For some Venetians, consent was not an issue, with widespread sexual violence. None of these avenues for disease transmission depended on prostitution.

Nonetheless, prostitution can hardly be ignored, especially in Venice, a city whose reputation as a haven for male tourists derived in part from its legendarily beautiful courtesans, the highly refined, educated women available only to the elites. The prostitute served as a complex symbol, representing sexual pleasure and freedom on the one hand and moral decay on the other hand, especially if she was a "diseased prostitute" infected with the French disease. These competing representations complicate discussion of the role of prostitution in Venetian sexual life, especially its role in disease transmission. But these representations do show, as the next chapter will discuss, how thoroughly embedded in Venice's literary and visual culture representations of the French disease became. As the French disease became embedded in Venice's social networks, so too did it become part of its cultural heritage.

2
The Suspected Culprits: Dangerously Beautiful Prostitutes and Debauched Men

During the 1550s, Antonio Musa Brasavola's (1500–55) theory of the origins of the French disease within the body of a prostitute enjoyed a certain popularity in Venice through multiple publications in the original Latin, as well as in Italian, translated and with occasional commentary, depending on the edition, by Pietro Rostinio.[1] The Italian language edition of Musa Brasavola's French disease treatise apparently reached a wide audience, with a version in 1556 and reprints in 1559 and 1565. After the French invasion of Italy in 1494, he explained, a most beautiful prostitute served the French troops. At the opening of her womb was a putrefying sore; the combination of the humidity and putrefaction of that "place," along with the rubbing of the male member against it, caused the male member to break out in ulcers. "And this illness began to stain one man, then two, and three, & one hundred, because this woman was a prostitute and most beautiful, and since human nature is desirous of coitus, many women had sexual relations with these men (and became) infected with this illness."[2] This beautiful prostitute was responsible for starting the epidemic of the French disease that was dispersed through not only "all of Italy, France, and throughout all of Europe," but also Asia and Africa.[3] The only region that escaped the beautiful prostitute's influence was India, where the disease was, according to Musa Brasavola, already well known, thereby making this woman the epidemiological equivalent of the "shot heard round the world."

This chapter traces the history of how ideas about the French disease, and especially about its origins, became incorporated into Venetians' literary tropes and iconography about the dangers of female beauty, prostitution, and undisciplined masculinity as the disease became endemic in mid-sixteenth century Italy. Because the symbol of a beautiful woman or prostitute performed significant cultural work in early modern Venice, the public associated the disease primarily, but not exclusively, with beautiful prostitutes. The theory that a beautiful prostitute who had served the invading French army accounted for the late-fifteenth-century epidemic of the French disease resonated with popular perceptions and reinforced efforts to control disease by placing certain types of women in institutions (as described in Chapter 4). "Debauched" men were also culpable in disease origin stories. Undisciplined as soldiers and unchaste in habits, ruled by sensual pleasures, debauched men upset the natural order by allowing themselves to be ruled by women or by enjoying themselves with other males. The French disease therefore became a symbol of the dangers associated with uncontrolled femininity and undisciplined masculinity. Although these narratives of the French disease's dangers built on earlier medieval and Renaissance literary traditions of disease, beauty, and danger, their popularity in the early modern period can be partly attributed to the moralizing impulses of the Counter-Reformation Catholic Church, the political and military failures of the Italian peninsula, and the impact of contagion theory.

Anna Foa's insightful analysis of early responses to the French disease showed how Europeans avoided blaming familiar scapegoats for the disease, as they did in the case of plague by tormenting Jews, by projecting responsibility for disease onto the "Other" and by using "reassuring *topoi*," notably the iconography from leprosy. Although leprosy was a frightening disease, it was nonetheless familiar to Europeans. By likening the French disease to leprosy as a form of Job's disease, Europeans found a way of diminishing the sense of threat the new disease brought. Foa argues that the French disease initially lacked an iconography of its own.[4] By the mid-sixteenth century, however, this situation changed. As the disease became endemic throughout Europe, Europeans responded by incorporating the disease into familiar *topoi* about dangerous sexuality and transforming these *topoi* in distinctive ways. Because of the impact of contagion theory, French disease narratives focused on individual culpability for the origins and spread of disease, although the city or country as a whole might suffer for the sins of the few.[5] More importantly, gender became central to the narratives and iconography of the French disease, with a strong emphasis on the role of women's bodies as the location of pathology.[6]

This chapter's purpose is therefore two-fold: first, to explain and describe how and why the French disease became endemic in a cultural sense in early modern Venice. A disease that is "culturally endemic" is one that becomes a common theme, image, or trope that resonates with the particular culture. Descriptions of the disease as originating within the body of a beautiful prostitute who served the French army served a complex role in early modern Venice by representing popular anxieties about appropriate masculinity and femininity and about military, political, and economic vulnerabilities. Second, I emphasize that early modern discussions of the origins of the French disease, especially vernacular medical discussions aimed at a wide audience, need to be recognized as influenced by literary *topoi* that linked the sexualized female body to disease. Narratives of French disease origins which focus on the bodies of beautiful prostitutes or the indiscipline of soldiers need to be understood as cultural products, even if they do form part of the medical discourse at the time.[7] Guy Poirer has made a useful distinction by referring to these narratives as "literary syphilis" that demand careful attention to the symbolic role of disease.[8] Venetians' obsession with dangerously beautiful prostitutes and dissolute men reveals more about their cultural preoccupations and anxieties than about the actual patterns of disease transmission and risk.

Origin stories as cultural products

The danger of female beauty was a common literary trope in Renaissance Italy, revised by Musa Brasavola and used to dramatize the vulnerability of Venice and the Italian peninsula to the threat of the French disease. As earlier social commentators on AIDS have explained, medical descriptions of disease, especially epidemic disease, are "always partly founded upon prior and deeply entrenched cultural narratives."[9] At first glance, Musa Brasavola's description of a beautiful and "promiscuous" original patient bears striking similarities to—as well as important differences from—the ways in which, centuries later, several epidemiologists and writer Randy Shilts would portray Gaetan Dugas, the Canadian flight attendant, as "Patient Zero" or the index patient responsible for the transmission of AIDS to dozens of North Americans on account of his physical attractiveness and sexual partnerships. Handsome and physically desirable, with piercing blue eyes and blond hair, his job introduced him to airline passengers that ostensibly made it possible for him to infect patients throughout North America. He was hardly the only gay man infected with this new disease, nor were gay men the only victims. Although Shilts also mentioned a Danish woman as one of the early victims of HIV/AIDS, it was the handsome and seductive Dugas who attracted media and public attention, largely because of the moral and cultural narratives surrounding male homosexuality and its alleged hedonism.[10]

Similarly, the "beautiful prostitute" story drew its narrative power from earlier traditions that linked women to masculine (and hence military) vulnerability. Because of the importance of the HIV/AIDS pandemic in shaping contemporary perceptions of sexually transmitted diseases, it is worthwhile to point out the differences between the historical representations of the French disease and more recent representations of HIV/AIDS. For example, the beautiful Italian prostitute was blamed not only for spreading disease, but also for having created the disease within her own body. She was never identified by name and could not have been alive (if she had ever existed) when Musa Brasavola's book was published, whereas Gaetan Dugas was very much alive when he was identified as "Patient Zero." While Dugas was a living individual who became enveloped in myth, the beautiful prostitute was generic and nameless, always enshrouded in mythology.[11]

As Paul Farmer has shown in the case of AIDS, origin myths about epidemics do far more than explain the biological origins of a pathogen. Origin myths locate blame for the epidemic within a wider geopolitical and moral framework.[12] Similarly in the sixteenth century, myths about the French disease became commentaries on the Italian city-states' political and military vulnerability after the Italian Wars (1494–1530) and of Venice's ongoing struggles with Turkish military power during the sixteenth and seventeenth centuries. Furthermore, the image of a beautiful woman had particular resonance in Venice (often represented as a woman) during the sixteenth-century, when a combination of changes in modes of representation, in medical theory, and in historical, political, and cultural circumstances coincided. Venice was not the only city where associations of the dangers of beautiful women with disease became popular, but these associations were more potent in a city that presented itself to the world in the guise of a beautiful female form.[13]

Musa Brasavola's theory was popular enough to be published thrice within a decade in the vernacular and twice in Latin in Venice alone, with other editions appearing in Lyons, Vicenza, and other cities. But his theory never edged out all other theories of the French disease's origins. The popular empiric Leonardo Fioravanti, for example, entered the debate in 1561 with his own theory of the disease's origins: cannibalism practiced by the desperate French army spawned the disease.[14] The French disease continued to inspire speculation about its origins, partly because it originated in recent, historical time, but more importantly because the late fifteenth century epidemic represented a turning point in Italy's history. Once a collection of independent city-states, the Italian peninsula was now under the sway of foreign nations, with the precarious exception of Venice, still independent but no longer as powerful as before. During the mid-sixteenth century, as intellectuals tried to make sense of Italy's military decline, they focused on the French invasion of Italy and the disease named after this event.

Not all medical treatises attempted to explain the disease's origins, however: Niccolò Massa, for example, avoided discussion of origins in his Italian translation of his Latin treatise, but his book did not enjoy the popularity of either Musa Brasavola's or Fioravanti's, with only one edition published in Venice.[15] Certainly some readers only wanted practical advice on how to cope with their illness (see Chapter 3 on books of secrets), but a more broad ranging intellectual curiosity, including speculation about disease origins and its possible ties to the French invasion, may have sold more copies than practical advice alone. Musa Brasavola's work was the only vernacular book devoted exclusively to the French disease of the mid-sixteenth century to go through multiple reprints.

Italian preoccupation with military decline helps explain the Venetian reading public's continued fascination with the origins of this disease as late as the 1560s, when the French invasion was no longer a living memory but an historical event. Contagion theory provided the medical reasoning to explain how a single individual could be responsible for a pandemic of the French disease, but medical theories alone do not explain why doctors and the reading public were so captivated by the idea of a most beautiful prostitute as Patient Zero. Why a prostitute and not a soldier? And why an extremely beautiful prostitute? Medical ideas developed in dynamic relationship with other ideas, and were also influenced by the rich visual imagery of late Renaissance Venice, which, especially in the work of Titian, produced numerous representations of female beauty.

Venice as a dangerously beautiful woman

Although Musa Brasavola's idea that the French disease epidemic originated within the body of a beautiful prostitute built on longstanding traditions linking women's bodies to disease and disorder, the connection between prostitution and the French disease was not immediately apparent to the earliest observers of the late fifteenth-century epidemic. Of the earliest chronicles written by non-medical observers of the 1490s epidemic, gathered and published by the nineteenth-century historian Alfonso Corradi, none makes mention of a prostitute as the origin of disease.[16] Most blamed the invading French army for the disease, such as the Florentine chronicler Parenti, for example, who described the disease as new in 1496 and yet already extended through all parts of the world.[17] Prostitutes were curiously absent from these early accounts, save for the occasional reference to their being among the infected as well. When these early writers discussed the disease's origins, they usually ignored how the disease itself originated and focused their blame on the French army and its leader, Charles VIII.

Only two early commentators mentioned prostitutes or loose women in association with the French disease, but they did not construct a theory of the disease's origins as lying within a particular woman's body nor discuss female beauty. A chronicler from Bologna, Fileno dalle Tuate, remarked about the French disease that "there was no real remedy, except to let it run its course and it was found that women had it in their private parts (*in la natura*) and because of this many prostitutes were banished from Bologna and from Ferrara and other places."[18] Fileno held women accountable for this disease, and punished prostitutes by expelling them from the city. Similarly, a writer from Ferrara explained that the disease arose from men having had sexual relations with "dirty women."[19] The two writers were building on a longstanding association between women's bodies and disease that could be found in Galen's writings and was expanded through centuries of medieval commentaries. The association between femininity and disease was already present in Western medical literature.[20] The notion that a single, beautiful woman could cause an epidemic that would affect most of the known world was, however, relatively new, and developed from the combined influence of the New World discoveries, the Counter Reformation, and new medical trends during the sixteenth century.

Because the city was surrounded by water rather than walls, Venice appeared to be, in the words of Luigi Groto, a "new Venus born naked in the midst of the sea" and simultaneously an uncorrupted virgin, unconquered by foreigners.[21] Generations of foreigners have been fascinated with Venice's alluring but apparently unconquerable beauty. During the seventeenth century, James Howell wrote perhaps the most famous example of this association between Venice, female beauty, desire, and vulnerability:

> Could any State on Earth Immortal be,
> Venice by her rare Government is She;
> Venice great Neptunes still a Mayd,
> Though by the warrlikst Potentats assayd,
> Yet She retains her Virgin-waters pure,
> Nor any Forren mixture can endure;
> Though Syren-like on Shore and Sea, Her Face
> Enchants all those whom once She doth embrace;

> Nor is there any can Her bewty prize
> But he who hath beheld her with his Eyes:
> Those following Leaves display, if well observd,
> How she so long her Maydenhead preservd,
> How for sound prudence She still bore the Bell,
> Whence may be drawn this high-fetchd parallel,
> Venus and Venice are Great Queens in their degree,
> Venus is Queen of Love, Venice of Policie.[22]

Although Howell celebrates Venice's long-preserved maidenhood, his writings also convey the sense of how fragile that maidenhood could be: Venice's beauty was a tempting prize to her many aggressive suitors. The polysemy of the "beautiful woman" provided fertile ground for Venice's admirers to praise the city's virtues, acknowledging its commercial success as an independent Republic (suggested by Venus) as well as its stability and ability to resist conquest (suggested by the Virgin).

The symbolic association between Venice and Venus became troubling to Venice's admirers during the 1570s, as Jutta Sperling argues. First, the Venetian patriciate turned away from sea trade in favor of land investments, thereby making Venus's associations with sea-borne commerce less meaningful as an icon. Second, the devastating plague of 1575–7 brought a new wave of accusations against prostitutes, whose bodies had already been associated with the French disease and increasingly became identified with the plague as well. Many regarded the plague as a punishment for the debauchery of prostitution.[23] Venus's sensuality made her a troubling symbol during an era that increasingly associated beautiful women's sexuality with disease and punishment.

In the hands of satirists and critics of Venice, the "beautiful woman" that represented Venice's strengths could just as easily stand for the city's weaknesses. Venice's reputation for internal political stability and resistance to conquest and foreign rule were legendary. The "myth of Venice," the set of beliefs that both encapsulated and celebrated Venice's alleged political harmony and freedom from conquest, reached its mature form during the sixteenth century, notably in the writings of Gasparo Contarini and foreign visitors. The opposing "anti-myth of Venice" also found full expression during the sixteenth century in the hands of no less than Machiavelli, who condemned Venice's aristocracy for its "effeminate" decadence and its military defeat during the Italian Wars at the 1509 battle of Agnadello.[24] One of the most potent symbols was the image of Venice as a courtesan, which could represent liberty to Venice's admirers but moral disruption, corruption, and greed to

Venice's critics.[25] John Eglin has persuasively argued that the myth and counter-myth of Venice functioned less as polarized opinions about Venice, but rather suggested a certain ambivalence; images of the admirable, independent republic shaded into the images of a city filled with intrigue and rampant with vice.[26] Foreign travelers purchased images of Venice as a woman in emblem books and single sheets. In contrast to images sold in Rome and other cities, Venice was represented only by female figures, in particular the Venetian dogaressa (wife of the doge, the highest elected official in the Republic), the Veiled Virgin, and the Courtesan, a trio that represented the republic, chastity, and liberty in a way that simultaneously suggested ambivalence toward these values.[27] These images circulated throughout Europe, reinforcing the association between Venice, the female body, and feminine chastity/sexuality. Even the images of a chaste virgin Venice invited spectators to imagine the symbolic opposite, the sensual Courtesan.[28]

The potential danger of beautiful women was a common theme in Renaissance literature and art, which took on additional associations during the sixteenth century as the French disease was added to the list of dangers. The link between female beauty and danger had its roots in the Jewish and Christian traditions, with stories about temptresses—Eve, Delilah, and even the heroine Judith—who brought about the downfall of men. Renaissance writers and artists built on these traditions and incorporated their own anxieties about beauty, which were later reinforced during the Counter Reformation. As Brian Steele has argued, women's physical beauty could lead a viewer to think only of passing, sensual pleasures, whereas the representation of female beauty in art could serve the more ennobling goal of reminding viewers of the timelessness and moral value of art. Titian, for example, painted representations of ideal female beauty, such as the golden-haired woman reminiscent of Petrarch's Laura in his painting *La Bella*, rather than lifelike portraits of identifiable women.[29] For neoplatonists, art could resolve the problem of "the ambiguity of beauty," to borrow a phrase from Naomi Yavneh.[30] In Tasso's epic poem *Gerusalemme liberata* (1575), for example, the beautiful, evil temptress Armida, who distracts Christian soldiers from their goal of conquering Jerusalem during the Crusades, is converted to Christianity, thereby chastening her destructive sexuality.[31] Beautiful temptresses were generic in form, all possessing the same combination of long, golden hair, black eyes, and fair skin that Renaissance treatises described. An ideal beautiful woman was virtually never found in nature; she had to be constructed from many different women, each of whom might possess beautiful parts. One woman might have beautiful hair, another beautiful shoulders or neck, and so forth, but ideal beauty seldom existed in nature.[32]

The idea that extreme beauty seldom existed in nature and was, therefore, almost a deformity or monstrosity explains the sixteenth-century association between excessive beauty and vice. Renaissance aesthetics emphasized the importance of harmony, balance, and moderation.[33] The humanist Agnolo Firenzuola described ideal female beauty as "ordered concord, akin to a harmony that arises mysteriously from the composition, union, and conjunction of several diverse and different parts."[34] Beauty and virtue were therefore linked in the minds of Renaissance Italians.[35] Beauty and good health were linked as well, especially since sixteenth-century doctors published books that combined advice for healthy living with advice on cosmetics, hair dye, and skin ointments. Giovanni Marinello, who practiced medicine in Venice, dedicated his *Gli ornamenti delle donne* (1562) to "chaste and young women," with advice on how to cure leprosy, heal scabies, and color the hair to appear more blonde.[36] The boundary between medicine and cosmetics, if it existed at all, was extremely fluid: beauty belonged to the realm of medicine as well as art.

Extreme beauty could upset the careful balance of symmetry and proportions. As the humanist and scientist Giambattista Della Porta explained, beauty was a sign of God's favor; extreme beauty, however, was often accompanied by vice. Because nature gave gifts in proportion, extremes of beauty were joined by a proportionate extreme of virtue as well as extreme of vice. An extremely beautiful male might be vainglorious and lead an army on an ill-advised expedition, such as the ancient Athenian general Alcibiades, held responsible for Athens' defeat in the Peloponnesian war. Extremely beautiful women all suffered from the same vice: sexual excess. The *bellissima* Helen of Troy was unfaithful to her husband, Della Porta explained, while Laïs was an extremely beautiful courtesan (from Corinth who lived during the Peloponnesian Wars) and Faustina the allegedly unfaithful wife of Marcus Aurelius.[37]

As the Counter Reformation became a more important cultural force during the late sixteenth century, a moral discourse on beauty overlapped with the earlier discourse on beauty and harmony. Beauty was not only useless to a woman, it was potentially damaging for a wife. Vain, spoiled, and easily led into adultery, the beautiful wife brought more damage than pleasure.[38] Popular proverbs from the early modern period also suggested a certain mistrust of beauty, such as "Beauty does not put food on the table" and "Every beautiful new slipper becomes a worn-out old shoe."[39]

Religious imagery often reinforced the association between female beauty, prostitution, and danger, especially in the imagery of Mary Magdalene. Sensual, even erotic, portraits of Mary Magdalene as a beautiful sinner linked feminine beauty with prostitution. A twelfth-century hagiography of Mary Magdalene described her temptation to promiscuity on account of her own beauty, which increased her vanity and made men almost blameless in their inability to resist her.[40] The sixteenth century witnessed a veritable explosion of paintings of the Magdalene, notably Titian's titillating paintings, which presented her with clothing barely clinging to her breast, almost inviting viewers to imagine touching her (see Figure 2.1).[41] As Paula Findlen has noted, contemporary viewers responded to Titian's paintings with feelings of sexual arousal. During the 1550s, Ludovico Dolce described his response to seeing Titian's *Venus and Adonis* as a "warming, a softening, a stirring of the blood."

> If a marble statue could by the stimuli of its beauty so penetrate to the marrow of a young man, that he stained himself, then, what must she do who is of flesh, who is beauty personified and appears to be breathing?[42]

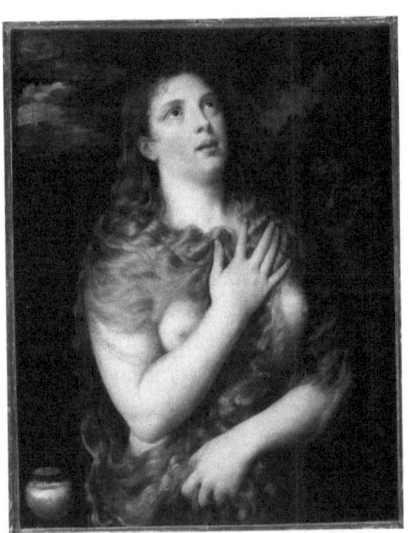

Figure 2.1 Titian's *The Magdalene*, ca. 1533, Galleria, Palatina, Palazzo Pitti, Florence, Italy. Photo credit: Nimatallah, Art Resource, NY

Dolce's reaction does not mean that viewers responded only to the sensuality of Titian's female images. As Rona Goffen argues, the images were never merely pornographic: the beauty of the images could inspire a range of aesthetic and emotional reactions, including the poet Vittoria Colonna's feelings of religious inspiration upon seeing Titian's representation of Mary Magdalene. Perhaps what Titian most effectively did was capture the erotic as part of religious feeling and imagery, rather than as separate and antithetical to it.[43] Sensual representations of the Magdalene coexisted in time with more sober images that depicted the penitent saint with hair covered and sombre visage, but the erotic images of the Magdalene never disappeared. The image of the repentant prostitute Magdalene became one of the central images of Counter Reformation Catholicism, partly a response to Protestant polemics against the alleged sexual degeneracy of the Catholic Church, and was directly linked to the French disease via the institutions for repentant prostitutes that developed within French disease hospitals (see Chapter 4).[44] Although repentance had long been one of the central themes of Christian thought, even greater emphasis was placed upon penitential practice during the late fifteenth and sixteenth-century religious revivals and reform.[45]

The association of disease with femininity also derived from European interpretations of the New World discoveries. By the 1530s, the French disease became the disease of the New World, a land that was represented in feminine form.[46] The idea that the New World was populated with sexually voracious young women was articulated as early as 1503 in Amerigo Vespucci's letters. Vespucci described the women as libidinous, gazing lustfully at the Spanish explorers and making their husband's penises swell to a large size for their own pleasure through the use of poisons, despite the potential danger to their husbands' organs.[47] As Mary Campbell sums up the range of European (male) reaction to the new land, "Las Casas wants to marry her to the Spanish crown, Ralegh to rape her, George Chapman to set foot on her 'broad breast' ... All the early explorers are drawn to the nakedness and comeliness of the Carib and Arawak women, who quickly become welcoming parties of nymphs for writers as disparate as the historian Peter Martyr and the poet Fracastoro."[48] By locating the origins of the French disease in the New World, represented as open, female sexuality, writers and artists encouraged the identification of the disease with the female body and femininity. Best known as the physician responsible for the renewed emphasis on contagion theory, Girolamo Fracastoro also wrote the epic poem, *De Syphilis*, in which he employs a narrative strategy that builds on, and ultimately reinforces, the symbolic association between the New World and disease, and especially between femininity and disease. Book III of the poem begins with a reference to a sacred tree "from an unknown world, which alone has moderated, relieved and ended suffering."[49] The tree in question was guaiacum, explicitly named in his text, well-known for its alleged curative powers against the French disease. The action of Book III unfolds on an island (Hispaniola?) across a sea, where the travelers from afar (Spaniards?) first "paid their respects to the unknown land, the native Nymphs and the Genius of the place, and you, gold-bearing river, whoever you were gliding with your glittering stream to your mouth by the sea."[50] The female nymphs without men, the promise of gold and easy riches: the imagery evoked the New World, feminized, with the simultaneous allure of sexuality and threat of disease.[51] Although Venetians themselves seldom traveled to the New World, they both produced and consumed an enormous volume of literature about the Americas. As "armchair travelers," they closely followed developments in the Americas, producing one of the earliest works on Columbus's voyages.[52]

Disease served as a convenient symbol of moral disorder for many early modern observers. As Deanna Shemek argues, the figure of the prostitute, disfigured by the French disease, became a vehicle for moralistic discourse in sixteenth-century Italy. "The Lament of a Courtesan from Ferrara", for example, was most likely written by a man between 1519 and 1530, but the narrator assumes the voice of a female courtesan in order to highlight the torments of the French disease with its attendant fall from grace and project blame onto courtesans, not their male partners. In the poem, the courtesan contrasts her previous beauty, which enabled her to circulate with the highest levels of society, to her current lowly status, unable even to sell candles to earn a living.[53] Other poetry continued with this theme, even suggesting that the icon of the Italian high literary tradition, Petrarch, contracted the French disease from his beautiful and beloved Laura.[54]

The idea that the French disease originated within a beautiful woman's body was potentially disturbing in a city that was so often represented as a beautiful woman in the form of either Venus or the Virgin Mary. Venetian writers also denounced courtesans as repositories of the French disease. As Margaret Rosenthal has argued, these denunciations arose from professional jealousy as much as from a sense of moral outrage. Dependent on the support of elites, male courtiers envied the advantage that sexuality brought to courtesans seeking elite patronage and relished the idea of their eventual demise due to advancing age and subsequent loss of beauty. For example, Venice's celebrated courtesan Veronica Franco endured countless insults from Maffio Venier, who wrote satirical verses denouncing her as ridden with French disease sores and a destroyer of good health, primarily out of professional jealousy.[55] Nonetheless, when she stood trial before the Inquisition on charges of heresy, her accusers (including Maffio Venier) emphasized the dangers of both moral and physical infection that her profession represented; "non più infetta questa Città" (she should be punished immediately so that she could no longer infect Venice). This combination of moral and physical contagion appeared in Maffio Venier's poetry as well, in which he described Franco as a woman "at war with good health" and a "sea swarming with illness."[56] Dishonorable sexuality and disease were interrelated for critics such as Venier: disease served as a marker of sexual and social disorder, in which women gained excess power through their beauty and promiscuity. Rhetoric about prostitution often was a discussion about the moral and physical health of society, thereby making it difficult to disentangle this rhetoric from the political and religious discussions in which it is embedded.

Prostitution: Disentangling the myth and the reality

Venice's critics seized on the symbol of the "prostitute" precisely because the city's visible and renowned courtesans lent plausibility to associating the city with loose morals. On the way to his incoronation, for example, the young Henry III of Valois (about to be king of France) stopped in Venice for ten days and visited Veronica Franco, an essential part of his tour of the city.[57] Not only was Veronica Franco legendary in her own time as a representative of Venice, but Venetian artists and guidebooks also indirectly or directly linked the city with courtesans. Titian's paintings still generate debate about whether they are portraits of courtesans;[58] and the famous tourist guidebook by Thomas Coryat highlighted the city's charms with careful descriptions and illustrations of a beautiful courtesan, her breasts temptingly exposed.[59] Of course, prostitutes and courtesans existed in early modern Venice and they both acquired and transmitted disease, but contemporary accounts of prostitution need to be interpreted critically in light of the symbolic weight the figure of the prostitute often bore, especially in Venetian iconography.

Prostitution had changed since the fourteenth and fifteenth centuries, making it more difficult to distinguish between prostitutes and other women because prostitutes were no longer enclosed in brothels. It is possible that reports of excess numbers of prostitutes are partly the result of their being more visible on city streets, rather than an increase in actual numbers. Throughout medieval Europe, cities owned or licensed public brothels in order to protect "honest women" by preventing rape and seduction, considered to have been an inevitable consequence of male desire which lacked an appropriate sexual release. Prostitutes who worked in public brothels were referred to as "common women" or "public women," available to all unmarried men, forbidden to refuse any.[60] Venice's history of prostitution closely followed the wider European model: following the logic of St. Augustine, Venice's great Council declared that "prostitution is necessary" in 1358 and established a public bordello, known as the Castelletto, located near the Rialto. In Venice, the city officials reasoned, a public brothel was particularly necessary because of the large numbers of foreign merchants and sailors who visited the city.[61]

Enclosing prostitutes within a brothel created a sharp division between prostitutes and other women. Even before the first French disease epidemic, public brothels began to close throughout Europe. In Venice, the public brothel fell into financial ruin and closed in 1460, partly due to poor location and partly due to failure to maintain its monopoly as the only source of commercialized sex in the city. The brothel met competition from private houses, despite the laws against them. The Venetian government was never effective in shutting out its illegal competitors in the sex trade, presumably because a few noble families were involved in running brothels and no doubt exerted pressure to avoid prosecution. With the collapse of the public brothel, according to Elisabeth Pavan, prostitution altered, and the courtesan emerged in the new, private world of the late fifteenth and sixteenth centuries: she belonged to one or very few men rather than to all men as prostitutes in public brothels had.[62]

The structure of prostitution had significantly altered before the arrival of the French disease in Venice, transforming the relationship of prostitutes to the rest of society. Although they were less socially isolated than previous generations of prostitutes, each of them typically had fewer sexual contacts, focusing their energies on long-term relationships with one man or a series of relationships with one man. This change in the structure of prostitution occurred throughout Europe, prior to or shortly after the first recorded French disease epidemics; scholars have described the closure of public brothels as a result of the changes in religious sensibility that brought about both the Protestant and Catholic Reformations.[63]

Both travelers' reports and parish censuses have been used to estimate the number of prostitutes in early modern Venice, but both sources are potentially misleading. All early modern estimates of the number of prostitutes need to be regarded with caution, especially since the word *meretrice* was often used to refer to any woman of suspect morals (including a single woman with one sexual partner who never exchanged sex for money). Marino Sanuto claimed that 11,654 *meretrici* inhabited the city of 100,000, a figure that most scholars have discarded as an exaggeration. In fact, Sanuto himself described the number as an "excess," which probably referred to the idea that a certain number of *meretrici* were necessary to protect the chastity of chaste women from unmarried men but an "excess" of prostitutes was problematic.[64] In 1608, Coryat reported larger numbers than Marin Sanuto in estimating the number of prostitutes at 20,000, roughly a century after Sanuto's estimate.[65] For a city of only 150,000 inhabitants, including males and females, children and the elderly, these estimates of the number of prostitutes defy all demographic probabilities. As discussed in Chapter 1, it is more likely that these numbers refer to single women, who were all too often conflated with prostitutes. In fact, parish censuses of the late sixteenth century reveal a much smaller number—only 213 prostitutes. Most likely, however, this number is an underestimate. Parish priests were responsible for carrying out the census, so some prostitutes may not have wanted to declare their occupation to a clergyman.[66] It is simply not possible to determine the actual number of prostitutes in Venice, given the limitations of the data, the broad use of the term *meretrici* to refer to various categories of women, and the way in which contemporary commentators used "excess" numbers to make a political or moral point.

Travelers' accounts provide an unusually rich source of writings about Venice that illustrate how the figure of the prostitute (as well as, for example, "the Jew") served as an allegory. Again, travelers' accounts often served as thinly veiled political commentaries designed to describe the strengths and limitations—the myth and anti-myth—of the Venetian polity and its mores.[67] Thomas Coryat's writings demonstrated to his English audience the importance of political liberty under Venice's balanced constitution,[68] but also exposed the moral hypocrisy of its Catholic institutions.[69] His narrative had less lofty goals as well. With a drawing of a bare-breasted courtesan and a detailed description of the "allurements of these amorous Calypsoes," his account was designed to titillate as well as inform his audience.[70] Sex sold books then as well as now. Coryat defended himself against possible criticism that he, too, was corrupt by claiming that although he visited a courtesan's house, he only conversed with her and tried, unsuccessfully, to convert her to a moral life. As he explained, "So did I visit the Palace of a noble Cortezan, view her own amorous person, hear her talke, observe her fashion of life, and yet was nothing contaminated wherewith, nor corrupted in manner."[71] Coryat's defense sounds like that of a famous American president who claimed to have smoked marijuana, but not inhaled. The presence of prostitutes represented the moral disorder of Roman Catholicism for a Protestant such as Coryat and a commonly deployed trope of English literature, especially after 1603.[72]

This kind of rhetoric illustrates the problems with a quantitative approach to the history of prostitution in Venice. It is difficult to ascertain the number of prostitutes in early modern Venice or anywhere in Italy because that information was not systematically collected in a way that would have been effective. Whatever Thomas Coryat was doing with his time during his six-week trip to Venice, he certainly was not conducting a statistical survey of prostitutes. Nor was anyone else. The tendency to exaggerate the number of prostitutes, partly as a political commentary on a particular city, occurred elsewhere in Italy, especially Rome, a city that shared a reputation for large numbers of prostitutes.[73] As these numbers are exaggerated, so too is the role of prostitutes in the spread of the French disease. As Deanna Shemek argues, early modern iconography of the French disease hides as much as it reveals by focusing on the role of prostitution. All fingers point to the body of the prostitute ("Mi mostrano a dito tutti quanti") in the art and literature of the time, thereby keeping viewers and readers from examining other means of disease transmission.[74]

Masculinity and the French disease

The symbol of the dangerously beautiful woman also pointed to another source of culpability for the French disease: undisciplined soldiers. In the wake of military defeat, and alongside a burst of renewed interest in "soldiers for Christ" represented by quasi-military religious orders such as the Jesuits, many sixteenth-century writers reinterpreted Italian masculinity as a source of vulnerability. Military discourse, especially treatises written during the Counter Reformation, reinforced the association between danger, female beauty, and undisciplined soldiers. For example, Ascanio Centorio's 1567 *Discorsi di guerra* praised chastity as a virtue for the soldier, giving the example of Scipio Africanus, general of the Roman army who brought Carthage to defeat during the Second Punic War. "A most beautiful young woman being presented to Scipio Africanus while he was in Spain, not only did he abstain from her, but he did not even turn to admire her, and ordered that she be returned to her relatives."[75]

The ancient hero Scipio Africanus was therefore able to do what the French and Italian soldiers of 1494 had failed to do: resist the temptation of extreme beauty. Scipio Africanus saved the Roman republic from conquest by Hannibal's legendary military brilliance, while the republics of Venice and Florence all but crumbled. Italian masculinity was not what it once had been during the glory days of the Roman Republic.

Writers like Centorio lamented that contemporary Italian soldiers lacked the discipline of their ancient predecessors.[76] Because of greedy leaders, the military had become an "ignominious market," "no longer worthy of that past glory," with soldiers weighted down in combat by carrying baggage filled with their own personal items. Here he underscored the prostitute's role in contributing to this moral and military decay, noting that armies were accompanied by "an infinity of whores": most soldiers even insisted on having their own prostitute at their very side as they fought.[77] His contemporaries needed to follow the example of the Turks and the Moors, whose soldiers he portrayed as more chaste. In mentioning the Turks and Moors as examples to follow, Centorio identified the principal threats to European, especially Italian, security during the mid-sixteenth century. Of course, by contrasting the chaste Turks with the incontinent European armies, Centorio and other military commentators played on Venetian fears of their vulnerability to the powerful Turkish army. Beautiful prostitutes not only brought disease, but they destroyed armies, navies, and, by extension, entire empires.

The idea that appropriate masculinity entailed chastity and sexual restraint did not win favor among some groups of males. Some sixteenth-century craftsmen, such as the skilled goldsmith Benvenuto Cellini, boasted of their sexual exploits with women, in which the acquisition of the French disease became a new badge of masculinity.[78] Conflict over models of appropriate masculinity intensified during the early seventeenth century in Venice, when the Venetian state came into open conflict with the papacy and expelled the Jesuit order during the Interdict Controversy of 1606–7.[79] In what Edward Muir has called the "culture wars" of the late Renaissance, Venice became the center of a particularly nasty conflict between the faculty and graduates of the University of Padua and the Society of Jesus (the Jesuits) which began in the 1590s and endured after the expulsion of the Jesuits. What constituted appropriate sexual behavior for men was one of the subjects of dispute. Known by their enemies as "libertines," the faculty and graduates of the University of Padua started the fashionable Accademia degli Incogniti (Academy of the Unknown), whose members wrote anonymous works satirizing the Catholic church, the Spanish, and conventional Christian sexual ethics from the 1630s to the 1660s. They condemned chastity as unnatural and advocated the expression of physical pleasure.[80]

One of the leading intellectuals of the group, Ferrante Pallavicino (later executed by the Catholic church), wrote a book *La retorica delle puttane* (The Rhetoric of Whores) in which he defends all sexual desire as natural, including same-sex desire. He rejected the Christian argument that only reproductive sex is natural and proposed a medical argument instead: sex is natural because retention of semen in the body is harmful and toxic, possibly leading to death. Pallavicino's espousal of sexual freedom was for men only, not women; he reiterated misogynistic themes about women's irrationality and encouraged relations with prostitutes. Women were merely sexual instruments for men's pleasure, according to Pallavicino.[81] Counter-Reformation moralists used the French disease as evidence of the errors of the libertines; in this case, disease was a punishment for men who frequented whores in their youth.[82] In many ways, the libertines were reasserting a freedom of expression, intellectual and sexual, that had been common in Venice a century earlier, prior to the Counter Reformation.[83] More ambiguous is Titian's 1560 painting of *Mars, Venus, and Amor*, in which a male soldier, shot by Cupid's arrow, has cast aside his armor to kiss and fondle the reclining nude figure of Venus. The painting depicts sensual pleasure as well as the soldier's temporary abandonment of arms.

Male sexuality was a contentious and fiercely contested issue in early modern Venice. Both models of appropriate masculinity, the Counter Reformation model of chaste restraint and the "libertine" model of free sexual expression, reinforced a fundamentally misogynistic view of women's sexuality, however. The sexually active women discussed in these texts were all whores (*puttane*). Men, however "undisciplined" they may have been, were never held responsible for the origins and transmission of disease, which was attributed to women's bodies.[84]

Seeds of disease and medical wonders

These literary tropes about the dangers of women's bodies, especially beautiful women's bodies, became incorporated into the medical literature of the sixteenth century in various ways. The sixteenth-century emphasis on marvels and monsters included speculation that new diseases could arise from the mixture of different kinds of semen or seeds, while a renewed interest in contagion theory rekindled interest in how diseases could be transmitted through sexual contact. Both of these trends in medical thinking contributed to the attention focused on the prostitute's body as a possible site for the origin of a new disease. Musa Brasavola's theory of the beautiful prostitute as originator of disease illustrates how literary tropes about the dangers of female bodies and medical theories about women's bodies converged.

According to Galenic and Hippocratic traditions still present in Renaissance discourse, women's bodies were considered to be colder and moister than men's bodies. Coldness rendered women's bodies more susceptible to disease, because heat could literally burn up any putrefaction within the body that could cause disease. In addition, women's menses were associated with uncleanness as well as with the transmission of certain diseases, such as smallpox, by contagion.[85]

Known as an opponent of learned Galenic medicine, the unorthodox Swiss physician Paracelsus made his own contribution to the association between a prostitute's body and the origins of the French disease in his 1536 *Chirurgia magna*. He argued that the French disease arose from the sexual union between "a leprous Frenchman and a prostitute with uterine sores."[86] Paracelsus's version bears a striking similarity to an earlier theory (1525) from Pietro Mainardi that the disease arose from the union between a Spanish prostitute and a leper.[87] Both Mainardi's and Paracelsus's theories invoke elements of contemporary cultural anxieties in naming both Spanish and French carriers of disease: Spanish conquest of the New World bringing disease along with its new economic and political dominance in the Italian peninsula, and the French invasion which unleashed the Italian Wars, in which the Swiss participated. Both rely on the older iconography of the polluting figure of the leper, in Paracelsus's case in a "monstrous union" with a prostitute.[88] Paracelsus was partially influenced by the renewed interest in monsters, marvels, and wonders of nature during the Renaissance, in which natural philosophers took an interest in explaining the natural mechanisms behind so-called marvels. Marvels included medical peculiarities such as a girl born without a vulva or a thief who survived hanging, and the appearance of new diseases, notably the French disease, while monsters appeared in a variety of forms, often mixing animal and human body parts.[89] Although Paracelsus's writings reached print only a few times before his death in 1542, he enjoyed enormous posthumous popularity in the 1550s.[90] An interest in describing and appreciating the wonders of nature, especially anatomical rarities, as part of nature rather than divine portents occupied prominent members of the celebrated University of Padua's medical faculty, including Realdo Colombo.[91] Although the University of Padua trained physicians from all over

Europe, its proximity to Venice—in fact, Padua was part of Venice's mainland territorial possessions—meant that it exerted tremendous influence on Venice's intellectual life.

The well-known lecturer in anatomy at the University of Padua, Gabriele Falloppio, linked the problem of prostitution to the French disease in ways that playfully invited his male audience to see themselves as "libertines." Falloppio's enormous popularity as a lecturer during the 1550s ensured that his medical theories would receive a wide audience among practicing physicians throughout Venice and the Veneto.[92] Falloppio made an explicit link to the problems that "beautiful prostitutes" presented to contemporaries, including medical students, in their ability to transmit the French disease. One medical student kept careful notes of Falloppio's lectures and recorded his advice on how to avoid infection should the students succumb to the charms of a beautiful prostitute. Significantly, the prostitute was described as being not merely beautiful, but "most beautiful," the same description that Rostinio used in describing his original patient (in Falloppio's Latin, *pulcherrimam*; in Rostinio's Italian, *bellissima*).[93] From the same University of Padua milieu that inspired the libertine movement, Falloppio espoused medical advice for libertines, linking relations with beautiful prostitutes to the acquisition of the French disease as a routine occurrence.

Similarly, medical images enabled physicians and medical students to indulge in an erotic medical gaze by viewing nude drawings of beautiful women. For example, Charles Estienne's anatomical pictures for an anatomical text published in the 1540s in Paris depicted women in erotic poses, displaying their genitalia as a form of foreplay, designed to titillate a male readership. It is unclear how widely available this text was in Venice, although the fact Estienne based his drawings on erotic images drawn by Italian artists, possibly even from Titian's workshop, suggests that French and Italian physicians and intellectuals borrowed freely from each other. The four scenes depict neoclassical figures of female nudes in the boudoir. The boudoir in each case is sumptuous, with tapestries, cushions, and vases, all suggestive of the courtesan's or Venus's luxurious surroundings as represented by Titian. In one illustration, the window of the room opens to an idyllic pastoral scene, reminiscent of the Tuscan countryside in the works of Renaissance painters such as Filippo Lippi and Petrus Christus.[94] Despite the use of male models for the images and consequent heavy musculature of the arms and legs, the anatomical images are nonetheless erotic. In one image, for example, the woman is reclining on her back on the bed, with her head thrown back in an expression of ecstasy, her legs splayed open in a pose suggestive that she is ready for coitus.[95] Erotic images of lovers in various sexual positions enjoyed tremendous popularity in Venice and throughout Italy during the sixteenth century, perhaps contributing to demand for erotic anatomical drawings as well.[96] Although the anatomical images did not specifically link women's bodies to disease (an image that might have revolted rather than titillated the viewer), they reinforced among their audience of male physicians and medical students a privileged "libertine" view of women as seductive objects, with whom sexual relations should be expected.

In 1559, Pietro Rostinio announced his aim to translate into the vernacular and add "many new things" to Antonio Musa Brasavola's Latin treatise on the French disease, an exaggerated claim since he changed only the front matter. As noted above, Musa Brasavola's 1551 treatise attributed the French disease to a prostitute with uterine sores.[97] In the first two editions of his book, Rostinio acknowledged his debt in the book's foreword to Musa Brasavola. By the third reprinting in 1565, however, Brasavola's name did not appear, as Rostinio's comments on the title page situated the book within more recent vernacular medical writings about the French disease, specifically the popular empiric Leonardo Fioravanti's treatise.[98]

Both Rostinio and Fioravanti were trying to reach a wide audience with their writings, but their tactics and methods were different. Fioravanti condemned the university-trained physicians and the elite culture which these physicians represented. Born in Bologna in 1517, he moved to Venice in 1558 and joined the ranks of professional writers, such as his friend and companion Francesco Sansovino, who criticized the Venetian elite. According to him, the problem with the medical elite was not just that they followed the ancient theories of Galen too slavishly rather than relying on "natural methods" of healing, but they had descended into the general moral corruption that engulfed the Italian peninsula, a place where flatterers, sodomites, and whores all thrived. "A creature of the Counter-Reformation," as William Eamon argues, Fioravanti "considered disease to be a form of physiological pollution analogous to the moral pollution that he witnessed in the world around him."[99] The French disease represented a fitting punishment for the sins of the people, which spanned the range from sodomy and whoring to lying and flattering. For him, the disease originated from soldiers' consumption of human flesh, a physical corruption in the body that produced disease and simultaneously represented moral corruption as well.[100]

Rostinio, however, did not distance himself from learned medicine. In the first two editions of his book, he capitalized on his knowledge of Latin sources to sell his book to readers, noting that he had translated these sources, and frequently mentioned Aristotle. In response to Fioravanti's commercial success, Rostinio adopted a different strategy in his book's third edition by dropping his reference to the apparently forgotten Musa Brasavola. Instead, Rostinio praised Fioravanti's book *Capricci Medicinale* as better than everything else written on the subject since Fioravanti clearly explained how the French disease originated during the French occupation of Italy rather than originating with the Indians.[101] Using this strategy of representing himself as a friend rather than rival to Fioravanti, Rostinio may have hoped to capture an audience sympathetic to criticism of elite medical culture. Nonetheless, his medical explanations of the mechanisms of the French disease were all a direct translation from Musa Brasavola's Latin text.

Perhaps the vernacular version of Musa Brasavola's theory enjoyed a certain popular success because it resonated with the public's perception of how disease originated. By locating the origins of the disease within a prostitute's body, Musa Brasavola had drawn on the complex visual and literary traditions that linked prostitutes to disease. In addition, Musa Brasavola promised to explain the precise mechanisms of how the disease originated and developed. To do so, he used another idea that had tremendous cultural resonance: diseases could develop from the mixture of semen within the body. The sixteenth-century fascination with monsters focused the attention of natural philosophers on how monsters were created. One suggestion was that monsters were created by the mixture of animal and human seed through the "unnatural" coupling of human and animal.[102] A mixture of many men's seed within one woman's body could therefore also be seen as unnatural and capable of producing a monstrosity in the form of disease.

Drawing on recent speculations about the role of contagion, Rostinio employed these ideas to explain how disease, once produced, could spread to others. In 1541, Venice had been the site of a government-commissioned consultation by the College of Physicians of Padua to explain the causes of an epidemic fever in the area. The doctors blended the idea of "seeds" as a kind of contagion along with the classical idea of putrefaction of the air as joint causes of this epidemic.[103] This metaphor of seeds was further developed by Girolamo Fracastoro. First published in Venice in 1546, Fracastoro's work on contagion was chiefly important for, as Richard Palmer has argued, his discovery of a language and image for the spread of disease that was more fruitful than previous images. The ancient Greek philosophers had articulated the idea of contagion, which continued to exist as part of the learned Galenic medical tradition during the Middle Ages. Medieval interpretations of how plague spread, for example, relied on a subtle use of contagion theory, showing how first the pestilence is generated in air, then disseminated by the contaminated breath or through pores in the skin through which contaminated air could escape and enter bodies. Air could also be emitted from a person's eyes when dying; a gaze could therefore also be potentially contagious.[104] Unfairly described as the originator of contagion theory, Girolamo Fracastoro nonetheless played an important role in the development of contagion theory during the sixteenth century: he systematized it within the body of sixteenth-century Galenic writings and revitalized the idea with a new metaphor.[105] Living things, called *seminaria* or seeds, could reproduce themselves and cause disease by spreading directly from person-to-person, by attaching themselves to an object such as clothing which enabled their spread over a small distance, or by traveling through the air and infecting a wider geographical area. Fracastoro's emphasis on contagion did not mean that he discarded the idea that changes in air and in the alignment of planets could produce new diseases, such as the French disease. His emphasis on seeds themselves, which shares the same root as the word for semen, is important for the ways it encouraged subsequent writers to think about the seeds of disease as the mixing of different men's semen in a prostitute's body to explain the origins of French disease.

The idea of sexual contagion also focused attention on individual bodies. Although medieval Europeans believed that, for example, lepers acquired their illness from sin, including excessive lust, the disease itself was said to arise from the imbalance of humors (especially black bile) created by that lust.[106] The idea of sexual contagion, however, did not arise until the sixteenth century, with important implications for the representation and understanding of disease. As Qualtiere and Slights argue, the French disease as a "sexually contagious" illness took hold of the imaginations of early modern Europeans in myriad ways. From Rabelais to Shakespeare, writers invoked the contagiousness of the French disease in a new discourse of blame: individuals could knowingly infect others. Prostitutes were particularly suspect and even subject to manipulation by others, as in Shakespeare's *Timon of Athens* (written 1607–8 but published in 1623), in which the title character seeks revenge on his enemies by sending a couple of infected prostitutes to spread disease.[107]

Musa Brasavola both borrowed from and influenced the broader cultural representations that linked the French disease to prostitute's bodies. For Musa Brasavola, the production and development of the French disease as a contagious disease within the body of a prostitute arose from the coincidence of several factors: environmental conditions, the mixing of different men's semen within the woman's body, the friction generated through sexual intercourse with multiple partners, the ulceration of the prostitute's uterus, and the thin-skin and therefore penetrability of the French soldiers' penises after coitus. How this new disease, created through climate change, could become a contagious disease, transmitted from individual to individual through coitus, demanded explanation. The French invasion of Italy had occurred during a period of great humidity and flooding, so this poisonous air was already present when the most beautiful prostitute arrived to serve the invading army. The friction of intercourse, along with the humidity of the vagina and putridity produced by ulcerations within the woman's body, was essential in transforming this poison into a contagion.[108] As Fracastoro had already explained, once the seeds of disease were present, all that was needed to make the seeds active was heat. Musa Brasavola alluded to the dark, hidden quality of the vagina by calling it a "cavernous" or cave-like place, in which a sufficient quantity of bad air had entered.[109]

Equally troubling were the thin-skins of penises, which rendered this organ vulnerable to infection. The thinness of the skin on the French soldiers' penises enabled the disease to penetrate the male member, ascend upwards through a man's body, enter his liver and infect the blood.[110] The object of sexual penetration, the penis, itself became penetrable, subject to infection. Through this vulnerability of the penis, perhaps especially in its flaccid state after intercourse, the male body became vulnerable to systemic infection. Musa Brasavola's concern about the vulnerability of the male member to infection was shared by other medical writers, notably the Spanish physician Gaspar Torrella (c. 1452–c. 1520), a longtime resident of Rome and witness to the initial epidemic.[111] Anxieties about the military vulnerability of Italy, invaded by no less than four foreign armies during the Italian Wars, were projected onto this description of the mechanics of the French disease's evolution. If the success of the French army raised troubling questions about Italian masculinity, Rostinio deflected these doubts by focusing on the vulnerabilities of French men's sexual organs. It was French soldiers' penises—and, by extension, French masculinity—that was to blame for disease, not Italian masculinity.

Although Counter Reformation discourse emphasized the importance of the male soldier's virtue and continence, no physician ever located the origins of the French disease within the male body. Newly reinvigorated Italian masculinity could perhaps prevent the onslaught of disease, if Italian men were up to the task. Meanwhile, blame for the origin of disease fell primarily on women. Regarded as humid and disease-prone, containing a mysterious womb, the female body carried the symbolic burden of disease from which the virtuous male soldier should protect himself.

Far from being dependent on the iconography of leprosy, by the mid- to late sixteenth century the French disease developed its own distinctive iconography as it became embedded in representations of gender, beauty, and danger. It is nearly impossible to separate ideas about the French disease in early modern Venice from ideas about gender. Italian masculinity suffered some loss of face in the humiliating wars that ended the long period of independence many city-states had enjoyed. The French disease became a symbol of military weakness and hence, especially for Catholic reformers, a reminder of the importance of chastity and sexual restraint. But there was never a consensus that disease represented the failures of Italian or French masculinity: competing conceptions of masculinity meant that for some men, the French disease could serve as a battle scar of a different kind, evidence of sexual conquest of females.

Considerably greater consensus existed on the meanings associated with female bodies and disease. In the hands of both Catholic reformers and libertines, in addition to medical writers and others, the French disease represented the simultaneous attractions and dangers of female sexuality. This association was, however, always negative: diseased women represented a warning, never a triumph. In a city such as Venice, so often represented as a beautiful woman, the image of a beautiful female who exposed others to danger and disease had particular resonance. The association between the French disease and the beautiful prostitute was, of course, not unique to Venice, nor was "the beautiful prostitute" ever the exclusive representation of the disease within Venice. The French disease itself became a symbol that could evoke multiple meanings; skillful writers and artists deployed this symbol precisely because it developed rich layers of meaning during the early modern period. Vernacular medical writings need to be situated within this broader cultural context, because medical writers, often unknowingly, deployed literary tropes and symbols to describe disease origins.

Modern readers may easily find fault with the sixteenth century's double standards for men and women, but nonetheless be tempted to take these representations literally as statements of fact about risk groups in early modern Venice. Did the existence of female prostitutes explain why the French disease became endemic in early modern Venice? After all, prostitutes are a known "risk group" because they have multiple sexual partners. As shown in Chapter 1, the problem with this analysis is that it is too simplistic. Diseases can be spread in a variety of sexual relationships, licit and illicit, whether socially accepted or proscribed: focusing on prostitution alone draws attention away from other situations in which disease transmission occurs. Despite Venice's reputation as a haven for prostitution, the reality was more complex.

Just as importantly, however, literal interpretations of early modern representations of gender, prostitution, and discourse obscure insights into what these representations can tell us about sexual disease in early modern Venice. The rich imagery that variously associated the French disease with a beautiful female/prostitute, with undisciplined soldiers and debauched men, and with the horrors of the invading French army in the form of cannibalism and other transgressions illustrates how the disease became endemic to early modern Venice in a cultural sense. Each of these narratives and images employed the French disease because of the symbolic weight the disease could bear to convey the anxieties that early modern Venetians faced during the late sixteenth and early seventeenth centuries. Although it is important to be aware of the ways in which the French disease functioned as a complex symbol in early modern Venice, it was also, naturally, a disease that disrupted people's lives. The following chapter examines how patients and healers responded to the disease once it was no longer a new epidemic, but a familiar and even routine disease.

3
Stigma Reinforced: The Problem of Incurable Cases of a Curable Disease

In its epidemic stage, the French disease frightened Europeans because of its power to disfigure as well as its apparent ability to cause death, albeit more slowly and less certainly than the plague. Initially, however, its connection to sexuality was tenuous: the French disease may have been God's punishment for sin, but the sin was not necessarily sexual, nor was the sin necessarily committed by the individual who contracted the disease. As the disease became endemic by the mid-sixteenth century, its ability to inspire fear diminished while its ability to stigmatize particular individuals, regarded as sexually immoral, increased. Two crucial transitions had occurred during the sixteenth century: widespread agreement that the disease could be passed primarily (but not exclusively) through sexual activity, and belief that effective therapeutics existed to treat the disease.

Once feared as an incurable disease, physicians and the public alike came to regard it as curable and hence less frightening. As a curable, common disease, treatment and care of French disease patients became a routine part of the medical and institutional care provided to early modern Venetians. For some patients, the French disease was not necessarily a disturbing diagnosis, since it was potentially easily cured and, if treated quickly and confidentially, not a source of shame. "Incurable" cases became the exception to the routine and the focus of stigma; physicians pointed to the patient's behavior—predictably, a "loose" woman or "debauched" man, or a patient who did not follow the doctor's advice—to explain treatment failure and deaths from the apparently curable disease. At the same time, the French disease had entered early modern Venetians' lexicon of insults and slander: French disease accusations were used to discredit witnesses in court, for example. How could the disease be simultaneously routine and boring on the one hand and stigmatizing and shameful on the other hand? This chapter answers the question by explaining how the complex system of health care in early modern Venice differentiated between patients according to social status, wealth, gender, and, most importantly, perceived sexual history. Practices that created and sustained social stigma became embedded in the process of diagnosis as well as in the unequal system of medical and institutional care, which in particular differentiated types of treatment according to gender. This chapter examines the types of medical care available outside of institutions, while the following examines institutional care.

A curable, sexually transmitted disease

As early as 1497, a few healers claimed to have successfully treated and cured the French disease, including a friar in Orvieto who practiced blood-letting and used ointments and wine-and-herb baths on his patients, as well as the university-trained physician Gaspar Torrella, who adapted contemporary standard medical treatment for treatment of this specific condition.[1] Their contemporaries, however, maintained skepticism about their claims. In a meeting of three leading physicians at the palace in Ferrara in March and April of 1497, the three men failed to reach a consensus on how to treat the disease. Each emphasized his own theoretical approach to disease and the regimen of treatment recommended by that theoretical approach.[2] While the university physicians argued over appropriate treatments, unlicensed practitioners, who outnumbered licensed physicians, initially filled the void, with a range of treatments.[3]

In 1517, two Augsburg physicians reported the discovery of a treatment and a cure for the French disease in the form of guaiacum, a wood, known as Holy Wood in Italy. The news spread rapidly.[4] Guaiacum, obtained from the West Indies, fulfilled sixteenth-century expectations of divine justice: because the disease was believed to originate in the New World, God wisely placed the cure for the disease nearby. The wood was supposed to be ground to sawdust, then soaked in water in a ratio of eights parts water to one part wood. The water should then be boiled until reduced to half its original volume; the foam produced during boiling should be dried and used as a medicine. The use of guaiacum was also controversial, however, with the sixteenth century's medical controversies infusing the debate over appropriate remedies, including the renegade physician Paracelsus's rejection of any tradition rooted in the ancient authors, Galen and Hippocrates. He advocated treatment with mercury, which enjoyed periodic favor among certain physicians.[5] A few physicians argued that guaiacum had actually changed the French disease itself by weakening the disease; once the disease passed to someone else, it was an older, weaker disease, more susceptible to cure.[6]

By the mid-sixteenth century, it was widely accepted that the French disease was curable. Girolamo Cardano, the University of Padua-educated physician, reported that he had a found a cure for the disease known as phthisis, claiming that the cure was no more difficult than curing the French disease. Nancy Siraisi has explained Renaissance physicians' confidence in their French disease treatments as at least partly a product of their ignorance. If many of these cases were in fact the same disease as modern venereal syphilis, then physicians would have mistaken its as-yet-unrecognized periods of latency as a sign of a cure. Those cases that were not syphilis may have been other, less serious illnesses or infections affecting the genitals that may have resolved on their own.[7] In addition to these biological reasons for why the disease may have been readily regarded as curable, there are also social and cultural explanations. As I describe in the rest of this chapter, early modern Italy developed an interlocking set of institutions to regulate health and healing, so that patients had recourse to justice, as well as to different healers, if they failed to be cured. Because hospital administrators believed that treatment was effective, they assumed that returning patients had become re-infected, rather than not having been effectively cured in the first place.[8] In addition, if patients made use of the legal systems at their disposal, tried several cures, and still suffered from the same illness, their illness was often explained as a result of their own failings as individuals. Stigmatizing incurable patients helped protect the reputation of healers.

The discovery of these cures for the French disease actually heightened rather than diminished some anxiety, given that the disease came to be regarded as a punishment for sexual activity in particular and hence a discouragement for those thus inclined. Even the controversial erotic writer Pietro Aretino expressed anxiety about the potential impact of a cure for the French disease on morality. Best known for his *Dialogs* featuring a young woman's decision to become a prostitute as the most honest of all careers open to women, Aretino earned a reputation as something of a libertine. Writing from Venice in 1542 to Michelangelo Biondo, Aretino praised Biondo for his contribution to the repertoire of cures, explaining the joy he felt upon hearing the news, but ended the letter with an expression of concern. What will happen now, he wondered, to those who had refrained from the pleasures of sex out of fear of punishment from this disease.[9] The discovery of cures helped fuel fears that nothing would keep a check on sexual excess; patients with cases of incurable disease bore the brunt of these fears by being stigmatized.

These fears of sexual excess developed after physicians reached a consensus that the French disease could be transmitted sexually. According to early modern theories of the body, coitus rendered men more vulnerable to infection than women, who usually acquired the disease only through copious amounts of sexual activity. The corrupt vapors of a woman's uterus could infect the male member, while the uterus's qualities of being cold and dry meant that it was difficult to damage and required repeated intercourse to infect women.[10] Coitus was, however, only one of many ways (albeit the most efficient way) to spread the French disease, including sharing beds, clothing, and utensils. Medical responses to the French disease throughout the sixteenth century continued to draw upon the flexible Latin Galenist tradition, in which a single disease could have multiple causes. The ultimate cause was always God's will, with a number of more immediate natural causes: corruption of the air caused by planetary conjunctions, imbalance of bodily humors, or the consumption of harmful foods.[11] Medical theory thereby allowed a wide range of interpretation of the causes of individual cases of the French disease, allowing for "innocent" infections acquired through non-sexual contact as well as infections caused by copious sexual activity on the part of women. Medical diagnosis protected some patients from stigma while singling out others.

Preventive advice was selective as well, as young men were encouraged to engage in sexual activity while women were not. During the first initial epidemic (the 1490s), certain physicians advised that young, healthy males in particular should continue to enjoy coitus in order to maintain good health, since retained sperm could become poisonous; according to one physician, the sick should continue to engage in sexual relations. Several physicians, however, warned against the possibility of contracting the French disease through sexual activity.[12] By the early sixteenth century, Italian physicians advised men and women to wash their genitals after intercourse.[13] Later in the century, Gabriele Falloppio targeted his preventive advice toward men, recommending the application of a medication-soaked cloth to the penis after coitus in addition to washing. He offered no suggestions to women for how to avoid contracting disease, nor did any other major treatise aimed at women (see below).[14] Falloppio assumed that his young male medical students would engage in intercourse; prevention was therefore all about finding the means for men to stop the infection, not prevent exposure. Preventive advice reinforced the idea that sexual activity was a healthy and normal activity for men and that disease could be avoided through sexual hygiene; women received no such advice.

The production of stigma

In 1633, Menega Bindona, a bead stringer, brought Angelo Lippamano to court to sue for lost wages and medical expenses incurred after he had severely beaten her. Lippamano defended himself by claiming that her long-term disability was the result of the French disease, not the beatings. He could not claim that he had not beaten her, because he had already been convicted on that charge and served six months in prison. All he could do was divert attention from his abuse and cast suspicion on her character. Among the many diseases commonly diagnosed and treated in early modern Venice, from continuous fevers to worms to typhus, Lippamano chose the French disease, no doubt because of the stigma it evoked. To associate Bindona with a nasty case of the French disease was to associate her with prostitution. Bindona responded by denouncing his words as slanderous (*maledicezze*) and asserting that her reasons for suing him were clear, not to be muddied with his vain accusations.[15] She recognized his defense as an assault on her reputation, not a neutral medical diagnosis. Similarly, in early modern London, many patients diagnosed with the "foul disease" (as they called it) lost their jobs or their housing because of the damage to their reputations. To avoid the shame associated with this disease, some committed suicide.[16]

This non-medical case clearly represents how stigma operates in several ways. First, the target of the attack is a female bead-stringer, a marginal form of employment confined to women who were not allowed access to guilds and skilled labor.[17] As scholars of stigma have argued, the impact of stigma usually falls most heavily on poor and marginalized people who seldom have the means to hide their illness.[18] The word stigma refers to a socially discrediting attribute that varies from physical deformities, failures of individual character manifest in alcoholism or imprisonment, to the "tribal stigma of race, nation, and religion." Stigma must be nonetheless understood in terms of social relationships, not the attribute alone. As Erving Goffman explains, a college education would be expected and usual for a middle-class modern American, but perhaps a sign of failure for someone working in a low-income job that does not require this education.[19] For a woman such as Bindona, the

French disease would be discrediting, a symbol of both economic insecurity as well as sexual license deemed unacceptable in women. While a working class man might view the disease as a sign of masculinity, the same disease held a different meaning for women at the bottom of the economic ladder. Men also had to meet certain standards of socially accepted sexual behavior or they could suffer stigma. Being perceived as unable to control one's desires, or as dominated by a woman, or as obsessed with sodomy—all these perceptions could discredit a man: the French disease served as a marker of these failures.

The system of medical and institutional care shielded some patients from stigma while exposing others. In early modern Venice, as the last chapter showed, cultural anxieties especially fixated on the figure of the beautiful, promiscuous woman and the undisciplined man, whether a soldier or an upper-class "libertine." Social and cultural norms influenced the entire process of diagnosis, care and treatment, and prevention advice.

One way to avoid this stigma, especially for those who anticipated judgment from physicians and healers, was to try to avoid direct contact with them at all. People who developed genital sores were likely to suspect the French disease as a possibility, since this was one of the symptoms commonly described and discussed. Venice's thriving publishing industry catered to the needs of those who tried to treat themselves at home with books of medical "secrets" and recipes that contained items readily available from the local apothecary.[20] Books included both internal and external remedies, that is, pills to be taken orally, as well as poultices and unguents to be applied externally to sores. In addition to these books of secrets, often written by healers known as "empirics" because of their emphasis on having found cures for specific illnesses rather than explaining causes of illness, university-trained physicians also wrote for a wider audience. Female readers in particular were a target audience for French disease treatment, based on the assumption that they were too embarrassed to seek treatment. For example, the University of Padua-trained physician Niccolò Massa claimed that he translated his book on the French disease from Latin to Italian specifically so that women could read it as well and therefore avail themselves of treatment they might be too ashamed to seek.[21] His book's title made a direct reference to the French disease, however, thereby making complete discretion difficult. Sometimes female patients were not the target audience for advice on sexually transmitted diseases, but instead healers who specialized in treating female patients, namely midwives. Scipione Mercurio's treatise on obstetrics (the only treatise in Italian until 1721, first edition in 1596) warned midwives about the potential dangers of gonorrhea (*"Dello scolamento, ò Gonorea delle donne"*), which many women were ashamed to admit and seek treatment for, thereby risking death. Gonorrhea was not regarded as a separate disease from the French disease; hence it provoked the same sort of shame. In order to prevent unnecessary deaths from this disease, he provided advice on how to treat this disease.[22] Women may also have been more disturbed at the loss of physical beauty that often accompanied illness since beauty was regarded as one of women's principal assets. Although men and women suffered from disease in equal numbers, beauty remedies were targeted toward women.[23]

Books of medical "secrets" that combined household advice with medical recipes provided another way for women to self-treat and avoid direct contact with physicians and healers. In her 1588 book of "secrets," alongside advice on soaps that make hands soft and beautiful, and oils that preserve youthful freshness and beauty, Isabella Cortese also dispensed advice on how to deal with unsightly sores on the hands and mouth created by the French disease by applying a concoction of dyes and herbs mixed with the fat of a billy-goat, chicken, and pig. While waiting for her cure to take effect, she told readers to hide the sores on their hands by wearing gloves. Whatever damage the French disease may have done to a woman's beauty, she promised to be able to restore. She also provided a recipe for a pill to combat the pains and boils that resulted from the disease; this recipe combined some common plant-based remedies, such as terebinth (the turpentine tree) and agaric, along with snakeweed (bistort) and a type of hellebore (*"elleboro nero"*).[24] In London as well as in Venice, respectable women with reputations to protect helped fuel a large marketplace in French disease cures that could be purchased privately.[25] The existence of these vernacular books provides evidence simultaneously of how common and how stigmatizing the disease was for affluent women. Cortese's book indirectly reassured female readers that they were not alone by treating French disease symptoms as routine and easily handled, but also offered them a way to obtain treatment confidentially and without shame.

Stigma did not fall on women alone, even if female sexuality was more troubling than male sexuality for early modern Venetians. For example, a priest, bishop, or monk would want to hide a possible case of the French disease because of the vows of clerical celibacy. Other men may have had a range of motivations to hide the disease as well. Most books of secrets and popular medical texts were not specifically targeted to female readers, but presumably reached a general audience predominantly of men. Typically, these books included a range of recipes for varying conditions, so the buyer did not betray any personal information by purchasing one of these. For example, one book published in both 1526 and 1530 in Venice aimed at both male and female readers by providing information on how to determine if a certain man or woman was potentially fertile. Tucked away in the third section, after the sections of recipes for good breath, good singing voices, and clean white teeth, the author included a recipe to treat the French disease, along with recipes for a wide range of other conditions.[26] Another book provided a French disease recipe that included a variety of everyday herbs and substances, such as incense, chamomile, earthworms, and chicken fat, along with an occasional exotic ingredient, such as Artemisia dracunculus or tarragon, obtainable from the apothecary.[27] This information enabled a sick patient to self-treat without ever encountering a physician or popular healer face-to-face.

Failure with one secret recipe did not seem to dampen enthusiasm for trying another. One vendor of secret medicines flattered potential patients by claiming that his unguent worked on persons of "quality." Having obtained his secrets from the renowned physician Falloppio himself, this writer claimed, he had cured 100 patients who had tried the traditional remedy of guaiacum three or even four times without success.[28] The more stubborn the disease, the more exotic and expensive the ingredients became. Instead of just simple chicken fat, this writer recommended the fat of a badger, bear, and goose, along with the blood of a male pig, to cure the French disease.[29] Only persons of "quality" would have been able to afford these expensive ingredients.

Because these ingredients were common to other recipes for a variety of ailments, the patient would not have faced any embarrassment in purchasing these ingredients from the local apothecary. Only guaiacum was associated exclusively with the French disease, and that ingredient was available only at the hospital. For example, bear fat and pig fat were used to treat head wounds, while Artemisia dracunculus was used to treat chronic coughs.[30] Apothecary shops were an old tradition in Venice as part of its spice trade with the eastern Mediterranean. In 1545, the Venetian Senate took this tradition one step further by establishing its own botanical gardens in Padua in order to cultivate medicinal plants from Crete and Cyprus, as well as collect medicinal minerals.[31] Because the cost of various ingredients and medications was fixed by the corporation in charge of apothecaries (the *Collegio degli Speziali*), apothecaries had to find other ways than price to build their clientele and compete successfully against other.[32] It is possible that warm, non-judgmental attitudes toward customers were one way for apothecaries to build successful businesses, although it is difficult to establish whether that was the case. David Gentilcore has recently argued that the paucity of printed handbills for French disease remedies in Italy can be explained by the ease with which patients were able to purchase their own medications from a pharmacist's shop. Presumably, patients would only have patronized these establishments if they felt comfortable there.[33] In contrast, in early modern London, printed handbills for "pox" treatments abounded where it was more difficult to purchase medication directly from the apothecary.[34]

Self-treatment was therefore an option for those who wanted to keep their identities and diagnosis secret. But self-treatment did not always lead to recovery. After unsuccessfully trying several recipes at home to treat disease, patients were left with at least three other options: they could consult a licensed healer, consult a university-trained practitioner, or attempt to gain admission to the Incurables hospital with its subsidized access to Holy wood (guaiacum). If, in the unusual case that these methods failed as well, the patient and his or her family were tempted to suspect that witchcraft was the root cause of illness. Physicians provided expert medical advice on suspected witchcraft cases in which they inevitably explained treatment failure as the result of the patient's behavior, not witchcraft.

Licensed healers not trained at university

Most French disease patients consulted popular healers as a matter of course, in the same way that they would consult healers for a variety of ailments that bore no signs of stigma. Healers offered cure-all medicines, or medicines for routine problems like skin rashes, aches and pains, and ulcers. Of the three means of accessing direct person-to-person care—consulting a university-trained physician, consulting a popular healer, or seeking admission to the Incurables hospital—consulting a popular healer or a university-trained physician were safer choices than the hospital for protecting one's identity and avoiding stigma. It should be emphasized, however, that many patients were not embarrassed about the French disease or concerned about public exposure. For those who were, especially the nobility, women, and members of the clergy, popular healers offered several advantages to French disease patients. First, they did not require detailed case histories, so patients did not need to discuss their sexual histories, as they did with university-trained physicians. Popular healers treated specific diseases, not the patient as a whole. Second, popular healers often blended spiritual and natural remedies, thereby suggesting the possibility that illness arose from witchcraft rather than from sexual relationships. This possibility might offer comfort to a patient fearful of stigma and blame. Third, popular healers were themselves vulnerable members of society, subject to potential arrest and detention by the Inquisition on accusations of heresy. If a high-status patient from a noble or citizen family used the services of a popular healer, the patient was aware of his or her relatively greater social status and power than the healer. The power differential most likely shielded the patient from the risk of exposure by the healer. Finally, popular healers included among their ranks a few women; female patients may have been less embarrassed to be treated by a member of their own sex.

Patients did not, however, consult popular healers because they were seeking an "alternative" type of medicine, as is common in Western societies today. Despite the competition between popular healers and university-trained physicians, there was overlap as well, especially in healing practices. For example, popular healers often mimicked the kinds of remedies and cures recommended by learned physicians. Popular healers did not therefore create an "alternative medicine" based on assumptions about the human body and nature of treatment fundamentally different from the dominant medicine as taught in universities.[35] Nonetheless, popular healers did occasionally provide substitutes for other common medications judged to be too costly or having too many side effects. Mercury was a common treatment for the French disease in the mid-sixteenth century. Healers and the public thought the intense sweating brought about by mercury cleansed the body of disease, but patients disliked the salivation and loosening or even loss of their teeth. Hence, licensed practitioners sold mercury "substitutes" such as concoctions with juniper, which also produced sweating but not salivation.[36]

For many Venetians, especially men seeking treatment for a new case of the French disease, it was relatively easy and straightforward to purchase some type of medication from among the plethora of healers with remedies to sell. The French disease was regularly mentioned as treatable by a practitioner's special medicines, and the Health Board routinely approved applications for licenses to sell medications.[37] The Venetian government regulated the vast marketplace in French disease cures by requiring that vendors of medications obtain a license from the Health Board. To obtain a license to sell medications from a practitioner's "secret recipe," the Health Board required that the healer produce some evidence that the medication was effective by supplying the names of patients willing to testify that they had been cured. Although the Health Board did not record these names, it is nonetheless important to note that many French disease patients were confident enough to be willing to have their names mentioned publicly. Part of the reason these patients were willing to share their names is that first-time sufferers from the disease, especially men who were not clergy, were the least likely to be stigmatized. Applicants for licenses to sell treatments either specialized in French disease treatments alone, or more typically treated a variety of illnesses, such as the lone female applicant for a license to treat the French disease, Anzola del Sala, a married woman who also treated "ulcers in the mouth, continuous fever," the French disease and other "similar illnesses."[38] The majority of applications for licenses to sell medications were not, however, for the French disease, but for a variety of common aliments, including toothaches, pains, and worms. Most vendors of secret medications did not need to rely on the French disease to earn their living,[39] but a few depended on income from medications for this disease in particular.

It apparently did not seem a contradiction to the Health Board officers that the disease continued to afflict so many Venetians in spite of the proliferations of medications. On March 14, 1602, for example, the Health Board approved Davit Tribulone's application for a license on the grounds that his medications would cure "those who will be oppressed from the French disease, as much the new (cases) as the old in the present city of Venice."[40] Two brothers claimed that they needed to renew their deceased father's license for a cure for this disease because they owed their entire income to this powder, which "brought miraculous health effects to miserable sick people."[41] These records with their morally neutral tone suggest that the French disease was common, and that stigma did not necessarily fall on the first-time sufferer who was readily cured.

Patients in Venice turned to popular healers for a variety of cures because of their charisma and reputations for healing, not because they were less expensive than physicians.[42] A few popular healers built formidable reputations. Although not a French disease specialist, the healer Angela Refiletti, for example, seems to have cut quite a striking figure and is a good example of the attractions of popular healers to their clientele. One witness described the following neighborhood gossip about her, "They say that she used to travel by boat, and they say she dressed completely in silk, and that she traveled with great ceremony."[43] It was this healer's wealth, status, and apparent success that impressed the neighborhood, not her humble accessibility.[44] She had apparently spent 17 years in the Levant, where she learned about different kinds of medicinal herbs, such as rue and sage, from a "father, dressed underneath in white and on top in black."[45] According to one of her patients' husband's testimony, the couple chose her after they had already consulted the services of two friars, recommended by the wife's sister. The couple therefore sought a spiritual cure before a natural one. The friars claimed that the wife was not bewitched, but half-witted (*"scema di cervello"*), so they consulted Angela, whom he described as 35 or 36 years old, but whose surname he claimed not to know.[46] It is not clear whether the couple really consulted two friars first, or believed that they needed to tell the Holy Office this in order to protect themselves from accusations of heresy. Whatever the case, the boundary between natural and supernatural cures was a porous one for many Venetians, as they often hoped to combine the two approaches. The possibility of being denounced to the Inquisition for heresy, however, may have encouraged patients to turn to friars for spiritual help with illnesses.

Not all popular healers cultivated such an air of mystery and glamour as did Angela Refiletti. Orsetta from Padua, for example, described her profession to the Inquisitors in terms of difficult labor. "I live by my efforts and by my sweat; I medicate gentlemen, and Monsignors, and now I medicate a priest from Murano who is called 'pre Paulo,' who has an ulcer on his member."[47] These bold and defiant comments did not win any admirers among the Inquisitors, although they provide a glimpse of a courageous and audacious personality, perhaps part of her appeal to her patients.[48] Given her defiant tone, it is difficult to know how to interpret her comment about the ulcer on the priest's male member and her illustrious patients. It could be taken literally as a list of some of her patients, or as an indication of her desire to challenge the Inquisition's authority and suggest that she had well-placed patrons to protect her.

Apart from genital ulcers, a few healers specialized in treating the French disease, such as Maddalena the Greek and her husband Ottavio da Rossi, a surgeon from Genoa.[49] For them, treating the French disease brought risks as well as income: they were denounced to the Holy Office on charges of practicing sorcery. As Ottavio told the Inquisitors when asked why people thought he practiced sorcery, "I must explain that when one medicates someone who has the French disease, (people) believe that one medicates by bewitchment." His wife Maddalena, however, was quick to point out her status as a foreigner to explain why she was denounced as witch. "Because I'm Greek, that's why they call me a witch, also because I medicate the sick."[50] Learned writers often defended and encouraged the popular belief that healers could cause illness if they allied themselves with the devil. One popular treatise on exorcism, for example, warned readers that those who practiced sorcery and witchcraft often pretended to heal illnesses with natural remedies in order to hide their malicious acts.[51]

The French disease was common enough a complaint for popular healers to know whether they had the gift for curing it or not. Another popular healer, Helen la Draga, included the French disease among a list of her specialties, including fever, backaches, and headaches.[52] But Zanetta Compiliti explained that she had tried to cure the French disease and been unable to do so. When called to visit a sick patient, "I go and see if the illness responds to me, because the French disease does not respond to me."[53] Compiliti's statement illustrates how medical practitioners operated within a world where healing took a broad variety of forms: Charisma, a particular gift from God for healing, could be important in choosing a healer. Religious and secular approaches to healing overlapped, as patients sought spiritual, herbal, and medical advice, often (but not always) from the same healer.[54] By the seventeenth century, the French disease was common enough for it to be a routine part of the treatment offered by licensed popular healers: a minority of healers specialized in the disease, while the rest seemed to have tried to treat it. Failure to treat the disease was not a sign of any shortcoming on behalf of healers or patients, but simply God's will in distributing the art of healing certain illnesses to certain practitioners.

University-trained physicians and surgeons: Stigma and the process of diagnosis

Unlike licensed healers, university-trained physicians were more likely to blame patients, not God's will, for treatment failures. Seldom was there an occasion to blame patients for treatment failure, since, as mentioned above, the perceived episodic nature of the French disease gave physicians the impression that they had successfully treated the disease. As shown in Chapter 1, the French disease was seldom considered a fatal condition by the mid-sixteenth century, so deaths were often attributed to other illnesses. Although the French disease became a routine and common part of the practice of university-trained physicians in early modern Italy, physicians inadvertently reinforced stigma in the process of diagnosis and in explaining patients' treatment failure.

This inadvertent reinforcement of stigma happened despite the relative friendliness and openness of early modern physicians and surgeons to French disease patients. In Italy, physicians and surgeons were comfortable with treating French disease patients and some even specialized in treating this disease. Unlike France and England, where popular healers and "charlatans" seem to have out-competed physicians in attracting French disease patients because of physicians' discomfort in treating the disease, Italian physicians offered routine care to male patients mostly without moralizing attitudes, as long as the patient professed to have engaged in heterosexual sex.[55] Prominent University of Padua professors, including Gabriele Falloppio, Eustachio Rudio and Giambattista Morgagni, readily provided suggestions on how to treat the French disease (Falloppio even claimed to have offered preventive treatment to 1100 men) because they assumed or even explicitly mentioned heterosexual sex as the potential source of infection.[56] Morgagni may have crossed out his patients' names from his clinical consultation notes to protect patients' identity, although it is possible that this was done later.[57]

Italian physicians' perceptions of a patient's sexual history, as well as the patient's own descriptions, influenced the process of diagnosis. Although they were less moralistic than English physicians about relations with prostitutes, they looked for specific kinds of sexual partners or sexual behaviors as evidence for diagnosing the French disease. As Rostinio explained, "If someone has had relations with prostitutes (*puttane*), and decaying holes (*caroli*) appear in his mouth, and in his jaws, in his throat ulceration appears ... it is easy to cure, but no sooner does it go away than it comes back again, this man has the French disease."[58]

This practice of taking into account a patient's sexual history differed from modern-day practice because, in early modern Venice, the sexual history itself was part of the evidence that suggested disease, rather than simply a clue to assist in the diagnostic process. External, physical signs, such as the ulceration of the throat, were ultimately less important for an early modern physician in diagnosis than the internal processes within the body, which were invisible and difficult to perceive. The French disease could appear with different symptoms in different patients, with no clear sequence of symptoms or even clear duration. As Claudia Stein explains, "everything depended on the quantity of the disease-matter accumulated in the patient's body, and on his or her individual complexion and living conditions."[59] A sick patient could even show symptoms seemingly similar to the French disease, but the disease would then change or morph into another disease.[60] With such apparent instability of physical symptoms, diagnosis of the French disease depended heavily on an assessment of the patient's history, temperament, and current living conditions, which accounts for early modern physicians' interest in patient's relations with prostitutes or other sexual behavior to serve as evidence of, rather than a risk for acquiring, disease. Frequent sex with prostitutes increased the total quantity of disease-matter in an individual's body, hence making the French disease a likely diagnosis for a patient with this history. Rostinio and other physicians used the word *puttana* or *puttane*, which was not a morally neutral word, but the same word used in street insults and slander.

Prostitutes were not the only sexual partners that made early modern physicians suspect the French disease. Rostinio also said that boys could contract the French disease if they were molested by a man, and again the language was not morally neutral. "If a boy is molested by a dirty pig (*porcone*), and in his anus, and around his anus pustules appear, that cannot be removed without difficulty ... this (boy) has the French disease."[61] Physical symptoms alone were unreliable guides to the inner workings of the body, so physicians relied on reports of sexual behavior to guide their diagnosis. Although the physicians themselves may have been tolerant toward patients who frequented prostitutes, they were apparently less tolerant toward those suspected of sodomy. In England, sexual relations with a prostitute were frowned upon, but were considered better than being accused of sodomy with a same-sex partner. It is possible that some patients may have claimed to have visited a prostitute in order to steer attention away from suspicions of sodomy. If a patient protested that he had only had relations with his wife, the physician might suggest another diagnosis—or suggest that the disease had been contracted through another means than sex, such as sharing of linens, clothing, or drinking cups.[62] Tolerant or not, the emphasis on sexual behavior, especially "deviant sexual behavior," as a key to diagnosis opened the door for the rest of society to march in with their judgments.

Particularly difficult cases to treat also ultimately invited judgment of the patient's behavior, lifestyle, and habits. Initially, if patients showed no signs of improvement after signing a contract for a cure and taking the prescribed medication, they could bring their complaint before the *Giusitizia Vecchia*, the magistracy in charge of disputes with guild members and workers.[63] The patient Triffon da Perastro, for example, brought charges against Signor Basselli for selling him a medication that was supposed to cure his case of French disease in a mere eight days, but failed to do so. After taking the medication, Triffon claimed that his illness never went away, since the pains in his legs returned after several days.[64] The existence of these contracts for cures, potentially enforceable through the legal system, reinforced the perception that the French disease was readily curable through purchase of the right medications. In Bologna, one barber-surgeon, Antonio Bossi, actually sued a French disease patient's family for non-payment, although the patient himself had died. Bossi was apparently confident that his medications had been efficacious.[65]

Instead of pursuing legal recourse in the event of treatment failure, other patients followed a different path: they suspected witchcraft as the cause of their illness. Although most early modern physicians acknowledged the possibility that witchcraft could be responsible for illness, they emphasized natural causes of illness. This emphasis on natural causes inadvertently reinforced stigma against patients, since physicians focused on behavior within the patients' control, rather than the external actions of maleficent beings.[66]

Early modern physicians repeatedly warned that common people too quickly assumed that diseases were caused by witchcraft rather than natural means. Exorcists and popular healers were partly to blame, according to Laurence Joubert, the chancellor of the Faculty of Medicine at Montpellier, who in 1578 published the first volume of a book titled *Erreurs populaires*. In Italy, his work had impact on the Roman physician Scipione Mercurio's frequently reprinted book, *Degli Errori Popolari d'Italia* (1603).[67] In criticizing ordinary Italians for visiting popular healers and witches for all types of illnesses, Mercurio distinguished the French disease as being a particularly striking example of the ignorance and superstition of the common people. As he explained,

> almost everyone for every headache, and for any other illness, first goes to find the *maleficia*, or witch (*strega*), to be signed, and (only) afterwards to the doctor, and for childbirth ailments, for tertiary or quartan fevers, for wounds or dislocations, and even for the French disease, they go to be signed by these (who are) really witches.[68]

The French disease was the only disease singled out with the qualifier "even" (*infino*) to suggest that turning to witchcraft for a cure was more ridiculous with this disease than others.

In fact, Mercurio could explain incurable cases of the French disease in a variety of ways, none of them depending on supernatural causation. Since God often used illness to convert sinners to repentance, and to inspire them not to drink too much, eat too much, or have too much sexual intercourse (*troppo uso di Venere*), incurable cases of a given illness could be explained by the magnitude of a particular patient's sins. If the patient's wickedness exceeded the patient's natural virtue, then a disease could be incurable.[69] God did make physicians capable of curing cases of the French disease, partly in order to inspire patients to return to God through evidence of his mercy.[70] But physicians could not remove sin from the patient: if the illness arose from sin, then the patient needed to go to confession, not just see a doctor.[71] In addition to linking intractable cases of disease to a patient's behavior, he also implicated women in particular as the real source of disease. The real way to free people from the devil's grasp was not exorcism, he argued, but the removal of women from the world, because nearly all major sins are introduced by means of women, or by men who through las-civiousness adopt the vanity of women.[72] Mercurio's interpretation of the causes of illness was not merely theoretical: they were enacted in specific cases when physicians were called upon by the church and state to determine the cause of illness. The following examples illustrate how Counter-Reformation physicians applied this idea of incurable sin and the culpability of women to individual patients.

Incurable cases, witchcraft, and stigma

If the French disease persisted after natural remedies had been tried, then the patient, his family, and his doctor might suspect that witchcraft was the real root of his problem. In these cases, the patient had at least two possible recourses: to consult an exorcist, or to make a denunciation to the Holy Office. An exorcist had to determine whether the illness was caused by *maleficia* before he could proceed with the exorcism.[73] French disease patients who suspected witchcraft and turned to exorcists did not leave a paper trail for future historians, so we have no way of knowing how many patients tried this remedy. If the illness were of diabolical ori-gin, the exorcist did not need to know the name of the suspected witch in order to proceed. But some patients and families feared that a witch could continue his or her diabolical activities unless the person had been caught and punished. If a particular person were suspected of witchcraft, the patient or his family could turn to the Holy Office of the Inquisition to denounce the suspected witch and prompt an investigation. What the patient was seeking was a cure, which the patient believed could not be achieved until the witch had ceased his or her (usually her) activities. The Holy Office used physicians as expert witnesses in order to deter-mine the cause of a patient's illness, whether of natural or supernatural origins. Physicians testified in French disease cases that the disease was of natural, not supernatural, origin, and sometimes turned attention to patient behavior to explain treatment failure.

The four trials in context

Only four cases out of more than 1000 records between 1580 and 1650 involve accusations of witchcraft as a cause of the French disease. The relative scarcity of French disease cases in the records of the Holy Office is itself noteworthy, considering that (as shown in Chapter 1) the disease was common and widely spread throughout society. Although the Inquisition trials dealing with the French disease are few in number, the cases provide competing opinions about the cause of illness, thereby providing some insights into how the categories of natural and supernatural origins were delineated. Through the process of deliberation over disease etiology, the French disease became established as a disease of natural origin, explained by a patient's sexual history and moral character. "Incurable" cases of the French disease therefore did not undermine belief in the efficacy of therapeutic practices and remedies, nor spark widespread accusations of and condemnations for witchcraft. Physicians and lay witnesses successfully challenged accusations of witchcraft in regards to the French disease. The Holy Office did not convict anyone charged with making someone else sick with the French disease via sorcery or witchcraft. The deflection of blame for the disease from the alleged witch onto the patient played an important role in the association of stigma with the disease. Although the Holy Office inadvertently served as a mechanism of "disenchantment" in early modern Venice by focusing on natural origins of the French disease, the Holy Office simultaneously reinforced the social stigma attached to the disease by associating the disease with immoral behavior.[74]

The four French disease cases investigated by the Holy Office involved four strikingly different situations: (1) a nobleman, gravely ill with the French disease, whose family accused his former lover of infecting him through diabolical, not natural, means; (2) an impoverished woman, ultimately convicted of witchcraft, who stood accused of having afflicted Angela Castellana, a prostitute, with the disease; (3) a married woman's mysterious death, attributed to naturally caused French disease by a lay witness; and (4) a man who rejected his doctor's diagnosis of the French disease in favor of witchcraft. The cases cluster chronologically in the years between 1615 and 1625, perhaps as a result of Paolo Sarpi's codification of Inquisition laws in 1613.[75] Between 1621 and 1635, Prospero Farinacci published his five-volume work on criminal law, which was widely read by Venetian advocates appearing on behalf of defendants. Farinacci argued, among other things, that it was sinful but not an act of heresy to command the devil to perform acts within his power, such as the ability to cause illnesses.[76] It is possible that Farinacci's work had a real impact on the type of cases pursued by the Inquisition, especially those dealing with illnesses.

All of the four defendants were female. Witchcraft was a crime with a strong gender component: in Venice, like most of Europe, the majority (but not the totality) of defendants was female, specifically 70 percent for the Venetian Inquisition.[77] Men, however, were more likely to be accused of heresy than women, with even greater numbers of men accused overall than women. Scholars have therefore downplayed arguments that witchcraft accusations represented a form of mass violence against women in particular.[78] But it is widely agreed that gender played an important role in the nature and extent of accusations. In Venice, men usually stood accused of the crime of using magic for treasure-hunting, whereas women faced charges of practicing love magic.[79]

The four defendants included one citizen; citizens formed part of the city's hereditary elite, immediately below the rank of nobility. The other defendants all came from Venice's lower social order, known as the *popolani*. The background of the accusers and the sick was even more diverse, from prostitute to nobleman. More crucial than social background alone, however, is the relationship between accuser and accused. Witchcraft beliefs suggest that strained social relationships can be the cause of physical illness.[80] One of the major motives for accusing someone of witchcraft was the hope that person accused would accept responsibility, remove the "curse," and thereby bring about a cure.[81] Early modern Europeans often saw a connection between social harmony and physical harmony: they inhabited an intellectual world that emphasized the correspondences between celestial and terrestrial harmony, between the health of the state and community and the health of individual bodies.

The Holy Office of the Inquisition

Organized in 1542 by Pope Paul III, the Holy Office investigated cases of suspected heresy in response to the growing threat of Lutheranism. As an independent city-state suspicious of the Vatican's territorial expansion and influence in political affairs, Venice tried to protect itself from unnecessary papal interference in domestic affairs. Instead of allowing the Roman Inquisition to operate unfettered in Venetian territory, Venetians insisted that three of the six officials serving on the tribunal of the Holy Office were laymen appointed by the Venetian government. The original tribunal included three prominent Venetian senators and began prosecuting cases in 1547.[82] By the 1580s, the concern of the

Holy Office shifted from the prosecution of Lutheran heresy to the prosecution of witchcraft, magic, and superstition as the numbers of suspected heretics declined in the city.[83]

A generation of scholarship has seriously modified the perception of the various courts of the Roman Inquisition as harsh, uninterested in evidence, and ruthless in prosecution of the accused. On the contrary, witchcraft defendants standing trial before Inquisitorial courts fared better than their counterparts in other courts, especially those in northern Europe, because of legal safeguards observed by the Inquisition. One of the most important safeguards was the Inquisition's insistence that a witch's testimony had limited value in implicating others. While courts in parts of northern Europe used witches' confessions to arrest and prosecute others named as participants in witches' sabbats, the Roman Inquisition discounted this testimony as illusions inspired by the Devil. Second, the Devil's mark, a concealed physical marking on the body of a witch, played no role in inquisitorial courts, while in secular trials this evidence was often decisive.[84]

Venetian secular authorities succeeded in exerting some control over the power and authority of the Roman Inquisition in its territory by appointing lay representatives to the tribunal.[85] When a witch was suspected of having caused illness to a human being, proper inquisitorial procedure required a physician's expert testimony to ascertain whether the illness had natural causes.[86] In the public imagination, witches, or those suspected of being witches, were thought to have broad powers that included the power to heal and to cause misfortune. By the late sixteenth and early seventeenth century, the French disease had entered the repertoire of the popular healer, easily suspected of witchcraft and often female.[87] Because she claimed to be able to cure the French disease, it was easy for the public to imagine that she could cause it as well. But the Venetian Inquisition seldom exacted the ultimate penalty from those convicted: between 1587 and 1705, only two defendants were executed.[88] Healers whom the Inquisition judged to be orthodox Catholics often received no punishment at all.[89]

Andrea Marcello: Stigma and the irregular life of a nobleman

After a lifetime of successfully controlling convulsions, 40-year-old Venetian nobleman Andrea Marcello fell gravely ill in 1624 and did not respond to treatment. His "incurable" illness led his family to suspect witchcraft as the ultimate source of his sufferings: the most likely culprit, they thought, was his former lover, Camilla Savioni. At age 33, Camilla Savioni's looks had already faded. Described by her lover's brother, Girolamo, as old and ugly (*vecchia brutta*), Girolamo must have wondered how she could possibly have captured his brother's affections so thoroughly that he apparently had named her in his will as the beneficiary to receive possession of his house.[90] As the daughter of Venetian citizen Marco Savioni and widow of Leonardo de Foro, Savioni occupied a social niche one or two steps below that of her former noble lover: citizens formed a distinguished class who often worked as clerks and eschewed manual labor. After Camilla and Andrea's relationship of some 10 or 11 years' duration foundered, his family denounced her to the Holy Office on charges that she had practiced witchcraft by making Andrea ill.[91]

Renaissance Italians believed in the power of female beauty to lead men into temptation and potentially upset the social order through cross-class marriages and love affairs: love was a potentially dangerous and disruptive force.[92] In the popular and widely known romance epic *Orlando Furioso*, for example, the author Ariosto portrayed love itself as a kind of sickness that compromised a person's ability to reason.[93] For a woman past her physical prime, such as Camilla Savioni, to arouse such passions was exceptional, however: the only explanation Girolamo could understand for this surprising love affair was witchcraft. Renaissance literature was filled stories about ugly or plain women who used magic or witchcraft to capture a man's devotion.[94]

Girolamo's allegations of witchcraft extended beyond merely having bound his brother Andrea's affections to her. She had sickened Andrea with a fatal illness that, Girolamo alleged, was robbing him of his sanity and his physical health. A couple of physicians had treated Andrea for epilepsy and the French disease, but his health continued to falter, further evidence from Girolamo's perspective that his brother's real problem was bewitchment rather than natural illnesses. When Girolamo denounced Camilla to the Inquisition, he initiated a lengthy trial process that involved the calling of expert witnesses, including six physicians, to determine whether Andrea's illness was of natural or of supernatural, diabolical origin.

Andrea certainly was ill and dying in the summer of 1624. His younger brother Girolamo blamed Camilla for his brother's sufferings, which, according to Girolamo, began after he wrote a will leaving 1000 ducats to Camilla. According to Girolamo, Andrea's lifelong struggle with convulsions had been controlled through consumption of holy water. The convulsions and continuous movements of his left leg would cease after he consumed holy water, only to return later at night with strong heart palpitations (*"con gran battimento di cuore"*) and heavy perspiration (*"che grave stià perspirazione"*) that endured approximately one hour. The apparently temporary efficacy of holy water fueled Girolamo's suspicions that Camilla practiced witchcraft in hopes of acquiring an inheritance more quickly. Like other witchcraft cases in early modern Europe, close relatives such as Girolamo may have diminished their anxieties in the face of incurable illness by blaming a familiar person, who could be punished.[95]

Six different university-trained doctors testified during the course of the trial, at least three of whom stated that they had treated Andrea prior to the trial. The doctors thought that Andrea suffered from the French disease and epilepsy, but not all of them were willing to swear that the illnesses had no supernatural origins. Curtius Marinellus, a 64-year-old doctor of Venetian origin, stated that "I would not swear that his illness does not proceed also from supernatural evil, because the devil can deceive even doctors."[96] Another physician, 50-year-old Albertus Cerchianius, concurred with Marinellus about the possibility of supernatural causes. Although Andrea's epilepsy proceeded from natural causes, he also suffered from an "old" French disease that brought about two rubber-like boils (*gomme*) on his head. "And we, seeing the persistence of these illnesses and the variety of them, and some also extraordinary and infrequent," considered that there could have been injury from witchcraft, although there were no demonstrative signs of witchcraft.[97] These two physicians aligned themselves with one side of a debate that defended belief in the devil's capacity to cause illness. Nearly 50 years earlier, Fra Girolamo Menghi argued in his *Compendio dell'arte essorcista* (1576) that skeptics who traced illness to natural causes alone failed to see the real effects of the devil on the world. For Menghi, the skeptics "served as tools of a carefully planned diabolical ploy to achieve the unilateral disarmament of the human race."[98]

Other physicians who testified at the trial disagreed with Marinellus's and Cerchianius's analysis. Factors other than witchcraft could explain Andrea's persistent, incurable illness: his own failings as a patient, as well as his failings as a moral being. For the physicians who had treated Andrea, diagnosis, prognosis, and patient history were all linked. Giovanni Benedetto (*Jo.es Benedictus*), a 52-year-old physician from Verona testified on May 9 that a year and a half earlier, Andrea arrived at his house and "showed me his member that was completely full of hardened and ugly ulcers," which he treated. On subsequent visits to Andrea's house, Benedetto continued to treat his ulcers, as well as a tumor on his head, and warned him to attend to these sores, otherwise his case would become a "horrible French disease." Once the ulcers on his member got better, however, Andrea no longer stayed at home; Benedetto resigned himself to the situation and no longer saw Andrea.[99] Benedetto thereby identified a natural cause of Andrea's illness, specifically the French disease, and explained Andrea's failure to respond to treatment as the result of his failure to attend properly to his health.

By July, Andrea had completely "lost all of his senses," according to his brother. Girolamo was frantic. He complained that the trial was proceeding too slowly against Camilla, who had to be stopped before his brother died. Meanwhile, Camilla was kept locked up in the Casa del Soccorso, a temporary refuge for "fallen women," since the first of March, when her trial had begun.[100] At first she denied practicing any magic at all. The Inquisitors kept pressing her for information: they claimed they had heard from neighborhood gossip that she had been to visit a certain Agnesina, who practiced witchcraft, in order to get Andrea to return to her. Agnesina, a 30-year-old Greek woman, had herself been kept by a nobleman; after he abandoned her, she learned to practice love magic to try to make him return.[101] Camilla finally admitted to having "thrown the rope" several times, the most common form of love magic.[102]

Perhaps because she finally confessed, the trial did not turn out poorly for Camilla, despite the pressures Andrea's family placed on the Inquisitors. In addition, she benefited from the patronage of a physician. On June 20, a certain Francesco Marcolini, a doctor, paid 100 ducats to have her released from imprisonment during the remainder of the trial. His relationship to her is unknown. He submitted no testimony during the trial. On September 12, the Inquisitors finally passed a sentence on Camilla: she was allowed to go free. Her sentence's relative leniency probably resulted partially from her having made a confession, but physicians also played an important role in diagnosing the nature of Andrea's illness. Camilla's defense attorneys had brought in four additional doctors to testify that his illness was of natural, not supernatural, origin.

Particularly decisive was testimony from Vivianus de Vivianus, a 51-year-old doctor from the parish of St. Samuel, who made reference to Andrea's sexual relationship with a certain Cecilia Valiera in addition to other women,[103] and thereby concluded that the disease was of natural origin. As he explained,

it appears that the infirmity of this Signor Andrea Marcello was believed to be a disease that the doctors call epilepsy, great in itself, but seeing that this gentleman was also infected with *morbo gallico*, and seeing that he led a most irregular life, as regards to witchcraft we do not see the effects that for this illness we could suspect witchcraft. And we conclude that it was the natural illnesses of *morbo gallico* and *mal caduco*.[104]

Andrea's "most irregular life" figured prominently in his diagnosis. Even a woman who admitted that she had sought the advice of a sorceress and thrown the rope several times was not convicted of having made her former lover ill with the French disease through diabolical means. And even a noble family, with resources at their disposal to pursue a witchcraft conviction, was unable to make their allegations stick before the Inquisition. Less than three weeks after Camilla's sentence, on September 29, Andrea finally succumbed to his illness. His death was officially recorded as the result of epilepsy alone,[105] perhaps in order to save his family from the shame of the French disease. No evidence survives of the remainder of Camilla's life.

This case illustrates the process by which physicians and the Holy Office reached a medical diagnosis in seventeenth-century Venice. The possibility of demonic causation was taken seriously, even in the case of the French disease. Physical symptoms were noted and discussed. The patient's personal history, however, was just as important as the physical symptoms in reaching a diagnosis. The emphasis on a patient's personal history was part of the tradition of clinical medicine in early modern Italy, especially in the Veneto, where physicians who trained at the University of Padua often practiced. As Jerome Bylebyl has explained, the formal clinical teaching of physicians such as Giovanni Battista da Monte emphasized that external signs on the body and physical symptoms were only part of the process of diagnosis. Grounded in Galenic theory, da Monte looked for causes of diseases. External appearances were important clues to be interpreted, but the ultimate focus was the internal state of the patient. Clinical notes for a variety of illnesses included references to a young man's reckless way of life, another patient's "disorderly life," and a third patient, who earned da Monte's praise as "quite a prudent man for one of his class."[106] Physicians' consultations in late Renaissance Italy built on the medieval scholastic practice of bringing several doctors to a patient's bedside to formally argue about a patient's case.[107] The process of formal argumentation over diagnosis was therefore not a unique practice of the inquisitorial court, but a familiar part of clinical medicine as well. Just as importantly, this case illustrates the role that social stigma played in diagnosis and prognosis. Marcello's elite status did not shield him from allegations of an immoral life. Immorality could explain why the French disease, regarded as curable by doctors and patients alike, still claimed lives. Camilla's social status, although not as elevated as Marcello's, may also have shielded her from harsh punishment. Citizens were part of Venice's elite with personal and family networks linking them to doctors, lawyers, and government office-holders. What happened, however, when the accused was a poor elderly female healer with few, if any, of Camilla Savioni's connections?

The stereotypical witch: Bellina Loredana and the French disease

In 1624, Bellina Loredana faced charges in Venice of having practiced witchcraft by diabolically infecting a woman with the "French disease" in order to make her die a gruesome death. At age 70, Bellina exemplified the popular notion of how a witch looked and acted.[108] Elderly, unmarried or perhaps widowed, impoverished, she—at least in the minds of her contemporaries—no doubt suffered from envy: a perfect motive for practicing witchcraft. Worse yet, witnesses testified before the Holy Office of the Venetian Inquisition that for years they had seen her doing the kinds of things that witches did. She had baptized images, healed the sick (which suggested her power to do the opposite—to make the healthy ill), and used potions to bind a man's love to a woman. And, they added, she had given oil to a certain Angela Castellana, who had subsequently fallen so gravely ill with the French disease that she was reduced to begging for alms at the nearby Campo di Zanpolo. Bellina's trial lasted more than a year.[109]

On August 26, 1625, Bellina Loredana was convicted on nine counts of having performed "sorcery, magic, and diabolical operations." After spending one hour locked in the stocks in San Marco with a sign around her neck saying "For Witchcraft," she was conducted to prison to serve her three-year sentence. Three years in a seventeenth-century prison, where food was supplied only if the prisoner paid for it, usually exposed the prisoner to sufficient privations and not many survived. The odds of an elderly woman surviving this sentence were slim.

The reason Bellina received this harsh sentence, however, had nothing to do with the accusation that she had inflicted Angela with the French disease. Of the nine counts against her, not one of them involved Angela's death from the dreaded disease. Bellina's defense attorneys had successfully defended her on at least that one charge. She did not cause Angela's disease, they argued, not because it was not possible. Like other early modern Europeans, educated and illiterate alike, Venetians believed in the ability of witches to cause disease, even diseases that could be explained by natural phenomena such as sexual intercourse. Instead, they explained, she did not cause Angela's death because Angela was a prostitute. Prostitutes always died of the French disease: witchcraft was not necessary in their case. As Bellina's defense explained, Angela Castellana

> for her entire life was a public prostitute making her body available to everyone; and because of this she was already for many years full of the French disease sores (*gomme*) and other incurable diseases; where [at the hospital of San Giovanni and Paolo] she died miserably because of these aforesaid illnesses not for another [reason], as is usual for similar prostitutes and this is well-known, and obvious and thus the truth.[110]

Angela Castellana's illness failed the standard of evidence required by the Holy Office for conviction on witchcraft charges. The case is an example of how physicians' emphasis on behavior, especially sexual behavior judged deviant or excessive, inadvertently reinforced stigma against patients with incurable French disease. What about people who had led ostensibly moral lives? Were they blamed for incurable cases of the French disease? The next case, that of a faithful wife, sheds some light on this issue.

The doctor's faithful wife

In 1617, Margarita Marcellini died after a long illness which had endured for almost the entirety of her four-year marriage.[111] Her husband, a physician, had treated her with a number of medications to alleviate the suffering from her headaches, fevers, and open running sores over her body. Her illness proved intractable and unresponsive to natural remedies. He finally called in an 82-year-old priest, Ottavio Rati, on the belief that his wife was a victim of witchcraft. Rati found evidence of the practice of witchcraft on her bed: "quills of feathers wrapped up together, beans, grains of millet, some nails, and other things that I don't remember."[112] These items were common elements in the practice of witchcraft, so Rati had them removed from her bed and burned. But her illness persisted. Eight days later, her bed was searched again, and more items were discovered. A motive and a possible witch were discovered as well: a jealous sister who wanted Margarita's money, and a maid who knew how to practice magic.

One of Margarita's nieces, however, had a different explanation than witchcraft:

> I do not know that she was bewitched. I know very well that they were saying that in her house, but they did not know it. ... And as far as I'm concerned, I believe that it was that doctor, her husband, who was the cause of her death. He filled her up with the French disease. He did it just like he did to that other woman, that is, his first wife, who died of it also.[113]

The Inquisitors left no evidence of how they made their decision, but the suspected witch received no sentence and the final verdict was *nihil probatum*, or nothing proven.[114] The natural illness of the French disease provided a likely cause of death.

As Guido Ruggiero has argued in his careful study of this case, the testimony of Margarita's niece provides evidence that the body was already beginning to be explained in terms of physical propositions by common people during the seventeenth century. For Ruggiero, the case therefore provides evidence of the process of disenchantment.[115] This argument is supported by two other cases: a woman who testified that she thought her neighbor suffered from an unspecified illness rather than bewitchment, and a case in which the alleged bewitchment victim was said to have died of the natural disease known as the plague.[116] Nonetheless, these cases alone do not necessarily provide evidence of a widespread process of disenchantment, because illness represented the most difficult type of witchcraft to prove.[117]

Furthermore, read in the context of other French disease cases, other interpretations of Margarita Marcellini's case are possible. The doctor may have wanted to deflect attention—and social stigma—from himself. Margarita's niece's testimony also provides clues about the doctor's reputation in the family and her judgment about who was to blame for Margarita's death. As David Harley has argued in the case of seventeenth-century England, the ascription of guilt was an important part of the process of diagnosis and healing, especially among popular healers.[118]

Furthermore, a woman and her closest associates might also accuse a husband of having infected his wife with the French disease and seek separation on those grounds. When the noblewoman Isabetta Bembo requested a separation from her husband after six years of marriage, for example, one of her servants testified that Isabetta's husband kept another woman in the house and had thereby infected Isabetta with the French disease.[119] The French disease apparently provided concrete evidence of a husband's or father's neglect of his household: in one petition for guardianship of orphaned children, for example, the profligate father had allegedly infected his wife with the French disease, rendering one parent unable to work while the other died prematurely.[120]

The physicians who described the prostitute Angela Castellana's and the nobleman Andrea Marcello's disease seemed to be echoing the words of Mercurio in diagnosing their illness as a result of their immorality. More likely than not, ordinary people such as Margarita Marcellini's niece were aware that the French disease was associated with excess sin. She may have wanted to make sure that her aunt's husband, rather than her aunt herself, bore this stigma, and therefore mentioned that he had infected her with this disease.

Finally, the last trial is the briefest and occurred nearly 20 years after the Marcellini case. It is also the only case in which social tensions play virtually no role in producing the witchcraft accusations. The victim had only a superficial relationship to the alleged witch: the denunciation therefore focused on the victim's experience of medical failure, which led him to suspicions of witchcraft.

The patient questions the diagnosis: Domenico Querini

In 1642, 40-year old gondolier Domenico Querini refused to believe his doctor's diagnosis that he suffered from the French disease. "I was medicated only by a doctor for about 15 days and he came everyday, and he told me that I have the French disease, and I assured him that I did not." It is not clear why Domenico believed he did not have the French disease: because the disease had been cured or because he had never contracted it. Despite his disagreement with the doctor's diagnosis, he continued to be treated by him for pain in his shoulder. When his shoulder did not improve, the doctor suggested that perhaps he had been bewitched and should consult a priest. Domenico was suspicious of a certain laundress named Mattea who had access to his clothing and therefore the means by which to bewitch him. Although the Inquisitors found his case sufficiently convincing to try to track down Mattea, the case nonetheless ended abruptly, with Mattea never appearing in court.[121]

Unlike the other cases, in this case it was the physician who apparently suggested the possibility of witchcraft as the cause of the French disease, at least according to the patient's testimony. The patient may have been trying to protect himself by saying that he was following doctor's orders. Although many physicians expressed skepticism about supernatural causes of illness, it is important to recognize that not all did so. By implicating witchcraft, physicians and patients had an explanation for why treatment failed. It should not be assumed that there was anything cynical on physicians' part when they turned to witchcraft as an explanation for treatment failure.[122] Physicians believed that the French disease was curable. Within their system of understanding, it was reasonable to consider bewitchment as a possible explanation for failure to cure this disease. One reason for suspecting witchcraft in seventeenth-century New England, for example, was if medication did not work in accustomed ways or did not work at all.[123] Significantly, Domenico's case is the only one of the four in which the patient's behavior, or patient's sexual partner's behavior, did not come under scrutiny. The suggestion of witchcraft may have shielded Domenico from blame, although it is difficult to know from this abbreviated case.

As a commonly encountered, endemic disease, the French disease became a routine part of the practice of early modern healers. In Italy, university-trained physicians and popular healers alike treated many patients suffering from this disease. Despite its commonality, the French disease nonetheless potentially exposed its sufferers to social stigma. For many patients, stigma could be avoided through self-treatment based on recipes sold in widely available "books of secrets" using common ingredients purchased from a pharmacy. Easily treated cases that could be handled confidentially posed little risk to a patient's reputation, especially if the patient were male and not a clergyman. Women seemed to suffer greater potential risk of social stigma, due to sexual double standards of conduct for men and women.

Cases that did not respond to repeated treatment raised questions. Patients sometimes blamed health practitioners for selling them useless treatment and took their cases to court. Rather than undermining belief in the efficacy of available therapeutics, the legal system of recourse apparently reinforced patients' confidence in the system of therapeutics as a whole. Individual physicians or healers may have been scoundrels, but patients did believe that they could and should be cured of the French disease. The healers themselves often had a different explanation: university-trained physicians tended to blame the patient's temperament or lifestyle for treatment failure, while popular healers suggested the possibility of witchcraft as the underlying cause of disease.

Suspected witchcraft cases reached the Holy Office, which relied on physicians' testimony to determine the cause of illness. In early modern Venice, the Inquisitorial court found no one guilty of having used diabolical means to sicken someone with the French disease. The court's expert witnesses focused on the patient's allegedly immoral behavior as explanation for incurable cases of disease. An "immoral" life provided evidence in favor of natural causes of illness, not diabolical interference.

Certain illnesses were more likely to produce speculation about supernatural causation, but the French disease was seldom one of those diseases. As in the case of seventeenth-century New England, witchcraft was more likely to be suspected if the illness in question presented unusual symptoms which did not correspond to a known, natural disease, if the onset of symptoms was acute, if the disease was rare, and if the relatives were suspicious of witchcraft.[124] The French disease cases studied here provide evidence only of the last criteria, the suspicious relatives. The French disease was commonly—not rarely—diagnosed in early modern Venice; furthermore, treatment failure could be blamed on the patient's behavior, or at least on the behavior of the patient's sexual partner, as in the case of Margarita Marcellini. By explaining incurable French disease cases as the result of immorality, physicians were invoking the idea that the disease was sent as punishment from God. Unsurprisingly, Counter-Reformation morality held sway in the Inquisitorial court.

This chapter has recounted a somewhat ambivalent story. On the one hand, French disease patients could easily obtain treatment from a variety of sources. A simple, first- or even second-time case of the French disease, especially for an adult male who could claim to enjoy vigorous heterosexual activities, was routine and brought virtually no moral opprobrium onto the patient. On the other hand, the process of diagnosis, however, sorted patients into different categories, some of whom received less sympathetic treatment from medical practitioners. Because of the practice of carefully examining a patient's history and lifestyle, university-trained physicians emphasized the moral failings of certain patients as the cause of their suffering and illness. By describing incurable cases of the French disease as a result of the irregular life of a nobleman, or the inevitable result of a life of prostitution, the medical experts contributed to the process of stigmatizing the French disease and ensuring that French disease patients experienced shame at their diagnosis. By becoming identified with prostitution and immorality, a French disease diagnosis not only brought shame on the patient, but it became a weapon in the arsenal of insults that could be used to discredit someone.

The practice of interpreting incurable French disease cases as a product of natural causes, not diabolical ones, brought mixed results to early modern Venetians. Shame fell squarely on the patient, not easily deflected through an accusation of witchcraft. In contemporary South Africa, for example, accusations of witchcraft are one means of deflecting stigma from patients with HIV/AIDS.[125] In Venice, although the Inquisition protected the accused witch, no mechanism existed to salvage reputations smeared by association, fairly or unfairly, with the French disease. Women who contracted the disease and received treatment until "cured" could salvage their honor by entering a special convent, originally opened within a hospital that specialized in French disease patients, for a life of prayer and penitence. As we will see in the next chapter, institutional care in early modern Venice also inadvertently reinforced stigma against certain French disease patients by singling out females for moral reform.

4
Gender and Institutions: Hospitals and Female Asylums

Unlike the plague, the French disease did not send its victims to a swift death, but lingered, rendering people unable to work for months on end. By the 1520s, Venetian authorities could not ignore what had become a widespread and different problem than the plague. Unable to work and therefore homeless, hundreds of French disease patients took to begging in the streets to the alarm and disgust of the city's well-to-do residents.[1] As a chronic, endemic disease, the French disease therefore required a different kind of institutional response than the plague. While Italians created Health Boards in order to be able to identify threats of plague and quarantine the infected and exposed, the French disease required thinking about longer-term institutional responses, especially hospitals but also a variety of female asylums. While men were offered temporary medical and spiritual care in the Incurables hospitals, women were encouraged to undertake a lifetime of penitence. Efforts at prevention also targeted females, especially young, impoverished beautiful females who might be the targets of male seduction; these young girls were enclosed within another institution, the Zitelle, until adulthood, as part of Venice's broader response to the French disease. This chapter explains how special hospitals and certain female asylums became part of Venice's response to the French disease, a new response that distinguished between endemic and epidemic disease and that institutionalized gender norms and prejudices as part of the system of care.

Guaiacum and the Incurables hospitals

John Henderson has recently argued that the French disease brought about a change in the organization of hospital care in Florence during the sixteenth century. As a chronic, endemic disease, rather than an acute epidemic, the French disease required hospitals oriented toward the problems these patients faced. Throughout the Italian peninsula, Incurables hospitals were founded to cater to the needs of those suffering from the French disease and as well as from other "incurable diseases." In this case, "incurable" meant long-term care. Renaissance hospital administrators distinguished between acute, epidemic illness and chronic, endemic illness: Incurables hospitals filled a specific niche to care for chronic, endemic illness.[2]

In Venice, the public health office (the Sanità) officially responded to the problem of the French disease in 1521 because it had become a crisis: the numbers of sufferers begging for alms on streets and in San Marco and the Rialto caused concern for the sick themselves and the potential for contagion to neighbors.[3] The Incurables hospital was established that year. Long after the French disease was regarded as curable, many patients throughout the Italian peninsula continued to receive their treatment at hospitals named the "Incurables." Prevention of further spread of disease was a concern as well, since the sick often smelled bad, and putrefying air and stench were thought to be causes as well as consequences of illness.[4] The hospital's opening attracted attention throughout the city for its spiritual as well as its medical functions: converted Jews were baptized, and the hospital's noble governors, including the son of the doge, washed the feet of the patients. The hospital had no trouble attracting charitable donations during its first years, enabling it to expand from 80 patients in 1522 to 150 in 1525,[5] although the wards for long-term stays were not completed until 1572 and 1591.[6]

A major motive for seeking admission to the Incurables hospital was to gain access to guaiacum or Holy Wood, whose exorbitant costs prevented all but the wealthiest patients from accessing the medication except in the hospital. Incurables hospitals had the advantage of large scale contracts to reduce costs.[7] The Venetian hospital offered the expensive guaiacum treatment only seasonally in spring. In nearby Padua, access to guaiacum was rationed by lottery; it is not clear whether Venice relied on the same system.[8] Hospital administrators received a multitude of requests for admission, especially when guaiacum treatment was offered. Patients apparently brought beds and extra food with them in order to increase the hospital's capacity to treat patients.[9] In Rome, the Incurables hospital possessed a monopoly on sales of this wood (imported by the wealthy German Fugger family); apothecaries had to obtain a special license in order to sell the wood. A similar monopoly of Peruvian bark, which was supposed to be effective against fevers, led to a black market in the substance: poor patients sold the bark on the side.[10] Rome's expenditures on French disease treatment, especially wood, were formidable: in 1562, costs for treatment of 754 males and 300 females were equivalent to 1.3 percent of total papal expenditures for the Papal State.[11]

Two well-known male patients in Tuscany explained why they resorted to guaiacum treatment after first trying a variety of other French disease cures. In Tuscany, guaiacum was only available at the Incurables hospital. Agnolo Firenzuola, the Florentine writer whose works include a treatise on female beauty, claimed to have caught the French disease and tried a number of remedies, all of which failed. He followed the recommendations of one physician to rest, and of another to become active, to no avail. He claimed to have exhausted the entire supplies of a nearby apothecary in the process. At last, he tried the Holy Wood (guaiacum), and was immediately cured. Similarly, Benvenuto Cellini, the Florentine sculptor and goldsmith also known for his autobiography, described his own frustrations with finding a cure for the French disease. Against the advice of his physicians, he too resorted to Holy Wood, and was cured. He allegedly contracted the French disease, he explained, from a beautiful young female servant, thereby reinforcing the association between the innocence of male infection and the ultimate responsibility of females for spreading disease.[12]

Men were more likely than women to receive treatment at Incurables hospitals, despite apparently similar rates of infection, as discussed in Chapter 1. In Rome, hospital admissions data from the sixteenth century survive, while in the case of Venice only eighteenth-century admissions data survive. Both sets of data show that women constituted a minority of patients at these hospitals, accounting for less than 20 percent of all patients in Rome during the sixteenth century and between 26 percent and 30 percent of all patients in Venice during the eighteenth century.[13] The most likely hypothesis to explain this situation is how stigma operated more powerfully against female than male French disease patients. Boards of governors were less likely to be sympathetic to female patients than male patients since females were suspected of having been prostitutes, while females may have been less likely to seek admission to hospitals in anticipation of social stigma.[14]

Interestingly, in Venice more people were reported as having died from the French disease in the hospital of S. Giovanni e Paolo (10 deaths) than at the Incurables hospital (5 deaths), which specialized in the French disease, during a 24-year period.[15] Of course, at the Incurables hospital, patients would receive treatment for the French disease; death was therefore presumed to be from other factors. It is possible that these patients who died, all female, arrived too late to benefit from treatment; two of the deaths include the comment that the patient came in order to take the water (made with guaiacum) and that the patient had suffered from disease for a "long time."[16] Another also suffered from fever, while the remaining two were female servants with longstanding French disease cases who presumably entered the hospital in April for the seasonal guaiacum treatment, too late to avert their deaths.[17] All five of these deaths cluster in April, again suggesting that these patients waited for the arrival of guaiacum in order to seek treatment. Although physicians and hospital administrators alike believed that the French disease was curable, they also believed that treatment needed time to work. A patient could be too far gone to save. These few deaths did not undermine confidence in the ability of physicians to treat and cure the French disease.

Despite this perceived success in treating the French disease, death was nonetheless a relatively common occurrence at the Incurables hospital, due to its role as a repository for those suffering from incurable, endemic diseases. An overwhelming majority of deaths at the Incurables hospital were attributed to sores (*piaghe*), accounting for 438 deaths during an eight-year period, in contrast to fever (3 deaths) and other illnesses which claimed only one victim (such as smallpox or *variole*).[18] Acute, epidemic disease claimed few lives since the hospital was not supposed to treat these patients. "Sores" were a condition that was not necessarily identified with the French disease, but an indication of incurable disease. In 1794, for example, Angela Scarello was classified as having an incurable illness and sores, but no venereal cause for her condition ("*inferma insanabile e piagata senz'avere mai avuto cagione venerea*").[19] The hospital clearly included patients with a variety of conditions, as well as a group of approximately 200 orphans, housed entirely separately from patients, beginning in 1588.[20] Those who died at the hospital may not have been diagnosed with the French disease. Of those who had been diagnosed with the French disease, Venetian hospital officials expressed confidence in their ability to cure these patients. During the eighteenth century, for example, the hospital discharged five patients that were described as "perfectly healed" after their French disease treatment.[21]

Despite the promise of effective treatment, some of the ill were reluctant to enter the Incurables hospital. Covered in sores, they took to the streets to beg and were unwilling to go to the hospital. The Senate responded by offering a sum of 30 soldis for each sick person brought to the Incurables hospital.[22] It is possible that the hospital's semi-monastic atmosphere was uninviting to some patients. As John Henderson has argued, the sixteenth century witnessed a "growing harshness towards those who were regarded as undeserving" poor.[23] The atmosphere at the hospital reflected its origins as part of the religious renewal of the early sixteenth century.[24] It is also possible that the patients associated the hospital with death. Unlike the hospitals for acute illnesses, many patients did go to the Incurables hospital in order to die in relative peace and comfort. In 1524, for example, the hospital admitted the impoverished nobleman Bernardo Contarini to stay in a comfortable place, separate from the other patients due to his noble status, while in 1525, a 92-year old man was admitted, despite having no incurable illness, as an act of charity for his final days.[25]

The Incurables hospital provided a central meeting point for various Counter Reformation spiritual and charitable activities during the sixteenth century, including the Society of the Oratory, which focused on providing Christian education to all.[26] One of the principal ways for the hospital to attract donations (on which it depended for 90 percent of its costs) was to capture public interest through its vocal preachers and charitable acts, which were deliberately showcased, as in the public conversion of Jews.[27] Christian education extended to the hospital's patients. Patients regularly confessed to the hospital's priest, who could require that they appear before the Holy Office if their confessions warranted further investigation. Pietro de Bononia, for example, a 24-year old former soldier convalescing at the hospital for Incurables, appeared before the Holy Office to confess that he had eaten meat the year before on a prohibited day.[28] The Magdalene story was also presented to male patients in the hospital for Incurables during the seventeenth century, with emphasis on the heroic aspect of her story, since she used strength to combat sin. Unlike the eroticized Magdalene with long golden hair barely covering her breasts described in Chapter 1, this interpretation of Magdalene emphasized her "masculine" qualities of strength. The brothers at the hospital composed a musical play in her honor featuring Mary Magdalene as a warrior, capable of defeating all enemies.[29] Through a combination of ritual, visual representations, music and song, and direct preaching, hospital patients repeatedly encountered messages about the necessity of repentance. The combination of required confession, possible referral to the Inquisition, and thorough immersion in religious education and rituals may have made the hospital an unappealing treatment choice for no small number of patients. For whatever reason, a few patients wanted to avoid treatment at the Incurables hospital, although for guaiacum treatment the hospital seemed to have always had a waiting list and more than enough patients willing to withstand the hospital's strict regimen.

The French disease, female beauty, and female asylums

For women, entrance to the Incurables hospital was merely the first stage in what could result in lifetime institutionalization. Public perception of the link between women's undisciplined sexuality and the French disease influenced the social and institutional history of Venice by contributing to the dramatic growth in new institutions for women during the early modern period, especially the sixteenth century. Fears about the French disease were not the only motivating factor for the establishment of new female asylums, but these fears did provide impetus to the establishment of these institutions and, more importantly, influenced how society imagined as well as how it responded to disease. Ideas about the dangers of the French disease and its association with the beautiful female body became imprinted in female asylums' founding charters and subsequently influenced their development and role in society.

Two of the new female asylums, the Convertite and the Zitelle, originated within the Incurables hospital specifically to respond to the problems created by the French disease. These institutions embraced narrow definitions of women's problems by focusing on undisciplined sexuality, thereby inadvertently contributing to these institutions' failures to confront the French disease. Because these institutions provided highly prized, scarce resources and services—shelter, physical security, access to education, an opportunity to pursue a religious life, and, eventually, protection of private property—places within these institutions were in high demand among groups who valued these resources, above all the reasonably well-to-do artisan families. As a result, these institutions changed significantly over time, serving as resources for the aspiring artisan class rather than as refuges for *meretrici* or girls at risk of losing their virginity. By the seventeenth-century, even those *meretrici* who did find a permanent home within the Convertite may never have had the French disease, since approximately half were virgins and the majority of the rest were former long-term, usually exclusive (at least for the woman) concubines or lovers of a nobleman. The former could not have contracted the French disease sexually; the latter could have contracted the disease from their lover, but were less likely to have been exposed to disease than women who had multiple sexual partners, for example prostitutes. At least two of these female asylums, the Convertite and the Zitelle, became what Sherrill Cohen has aptly described as "custodial warehouses" for a variety of women with no clear institutional links to hospitals or the French disease,[30] while the eighteenth-century Penitenti maintained its close ties to the Incurables hospital. Although female asylums served various social roles, they continued to perpetuate the idea that undisciplined female sexuality—rather than the host of factors influencing sexual behavior that were discussed in Chapter 1—was the main problem underlying the spread of the French disease. During the eighteenth century, Venice's elites shifted their focus from female beauty to female poverty as the root problem for the spread of the French disease, but women remained the principal targets of moral reform.

The group of female asylums that opened in Venice and throughout the Italian peninsula during the sixteenth century are not solely a product of public reaction to the French disease. In fact, most studies have understandably focused on these institutions' ties to the fundamental and widespread religious changes during the age of Catholic and Protestant Reformations. In late-fifteenth-century Spain, for example, Franciscan mystics in Castile emphasized the importance of internal change, meditation, and self-control, especially in the face of worldly temptations, rather than formal study and assertions of faith, for lay people's spiritual development. The idea of *recogimiento*, or isolation and enclosure, developed from this Franciscan mystic movement. A variety of asylums primarily for females, including those for "repentant prostitutes," were founded in Spain during the sixteenth century; *recogimiento* therefore encompassed a "mystical precept, behavioral norm and institutional practice" all at once.[31] The founders of Venice's Convertite were also influenced by Spanish religious traditions, by Ignatius Loyola, who visited the Incurables hospital before he founded the Jesuit order, as well as by Gaetano Thiene (founder of the Theatine order) and the Company of Divine Love, a charitable association of lay people and clerics active during the early sixteenth century.[32]

Once it became clear that the French disease had become a permanent part of European life rather than a temporary epidemic, however, Europeans renewed their interest in institutions for penitent women in order to serve a new goal: control of the French disease.[33] During the thirteenth century, convents for "repentant prostitutes" (prostitution had various meanings during this period as well as during the sixteenth century) dedicated to Mary Magdalene opened throughout France and then spread across the Alps to Italy. Because they lacked an association with a religious order and were not considered to be official convents, these institutions struggled to survive. By the fifteenth century, many had closed.[34]

By receiving permission from Pope Leo X in 1520 to found the new generation of convents for repentant *meretrici*, which formally adopted the rule of St. Augustine, these institutions found a secure place within the church's hierarchy and institutional structures.[35] In fact, these institutions became so entrenched in European culture during the sixteenth century that they became a vital part of overseas empires in Spanish America and in Portuguese territories worldwide.[36] "Repentant prostitutes" (more likely unmarried women who had engaged in sexual relations) served as the first female colonizers in, for example, Portuguese Angola beginning in 1595. The governor of Angola arranged marriages for all of these women, newly released from the Magdalene houses in Portugal, thereby solving two problems at once: finding suitable situations for unmarriageable Portuguese women, and providing spouses of the same race for Portuguese men in order to maintain social distance between colonizers and colonized.[37]

In Venice between 1525 and 1542, a group of "converted women" remained within the Incurables hospital until they were able to move to a building of their own. In 1551, they received permission to follow the Augustinian rule.[38] Although the only requirement for entry into the convent (besides the willingness to follow the religious life) was having led a "licentious life" and therefore being a fallen woman, the nuns nonetheless quickly earned a reputation for beauty. The convent's governors, as well as the church hierarchy, regarded beautiful women as more vulnerable to sin than ugly ones. In making the case for why Isabetta Arrigona should be allowed to enter the Convertite in 1606, for example, the petition on her behalf explained that she was "both young and beautiful," and therefore not safe outside of matrimony or an institution. In fact, youth and beauty constituted the most important qualities that made Isabetta eligible for entry into the Convertite. She was not a *meretrice*, since she apparently did not engage in sexual relations outside of marriage; her brief marriage to her husband, Michel, to whom she had been faithful, had foundered (for reasons left unstated in her petition), leaving her few options to "live honestly" outside of convent life.[39] She was therefore seen as vulnerable: sexually experienced, and young and beautiful, vulnerable to her own desires as well as a temptation to men around her. Beauty thus gave an added edge to candidates who sought admission to the Convertite, even if they were not *meretrici*. This admissions process most likely contributed to the institution's reputation for beautiful women. For example, in 1581 the popular writer Francesco Sansovino claimed that the convent housed a great number of penitent sinners, all most beautiful (*"gran numero di donne & tutte bellissime"*).[40] By the 1580s, the convent enclosed more than 350 women, a number which remained fairly steady for the rest of the convent's history.[41]

The nuns' beauty was apparently what attracted the first rector in charge of the convent, Pietro Leon from Valcamonica, to seduce approximately 20 of the nuns and induce abortions in those he had impregnated. The apostolic nunzio Ippolito Capilupi reported in a letter of November 1561 that Lion confessed to asking the most beautiful among the nuns to undress and bathe in front of him "*che le più belle si spogliassero e andassero a bagnarsi nella cavana.*" Those who were unwilling to submit to his advances were sent to the convent's internal prison.[42] Prior to his public execution in Piazzetta San Marco in 1561, he wrote a confession, explaining that he had committed these acts because "we are all subject to fragility ... also I saw and knew about greater faults committed by others than what I was doing, it seemed to me that my faults were much inferior to those."[43] Hinting that he was powerless to control himself, Lion played to contemporary prejudices about the power of feminine beauty.

By concentrating on beautiful women, the Convertite invited significant attention (and some trouble) from Venice's men. In November 1624, for example, the priest Francesco Montenegro was forbidden from saying the Mass at the Convertite after he was caught having sent a portrait of a nude man to one of the nuns inside; just four years earlier, the priest Giacomo Zenoni was denounced for having sent love letters to nuns in the Convertite, as well as to nuns in two other convents.[44] Priests were not the only men who found the nuns at the Convertite tempting. Men stopped by frequently to try to talk to them or just catch a glimpse of them, which was difficult to do once strict closure was imposed in 1563. It is clear that some Venetian men viewed women at the Convertite as unique from other nuns and thus open to their sexual advances. Piero, a musician, defended himself on charges of unlawfully trying to talk to the nuns by claiming that he thought they were "women of the world," not like other convents.[45] The attention that the nuns at the Convertite garnered must have only confirmed the authorities' initial suspicions about the effects of beauty on public order and public health. Extreme beauty was best corralled. A subsequent institution, the Zitelle, actually made beauty an official requirement for entry.

The statutes of the Zitelle explicitly required that girls who entered the institution be beautiful, thereby reflecting and reinforcing contemporary anxieties about the dangers of beauty and its association with disease. Like the Convertite, the Zitelle owed its origins to the hospital of the *Incurabili*. After he came face-to-face with the French disease while preaching in the hospital's church, Benedetto Palmio wrote that he felt inspired in 1558 to found an institution to protect young girls from the eternal damnation that could be their fate should they fall into sin on account of their beauty. A house of refuge would "liberate from the danger of eternal damnation a certain type of virgin, who being very beautiful, and graceful" was at risk of losing her virginity due to the malice of others acting "contrary to the health and to the purity of the Christian religion."[46] The statutes of the Zitelle tried to ensure that only girls who were truly at risk of being deflowered—defined as "at risk" on account of their beauty—were accepted into the Zitelle. New entrants had to be at least 12 years old but not older than 18, healthy, and beautiful; the governors should be particularly attentive to cases of impoverished, very beautiful girls, whose own parents or guardians might be tempted to let the girl be led astray in order to alleviate the family's extreme poverty. Two male governors interviewed each prospective entrant to determine whether she fit the institution's requirement. Detailed notes were not taken on a girl's appearance, but simply the judgment of "*bella*" or "*brutta*" (ugly).[47]

The requirement that girls be beautiful existed in similar institutions in other Italian city-states: Bologna's conservatory of S. Maria del Baraccano (founded in 1528), for example, required that the orphaned girls they accepted be at risk of losing their virginity on account of their beauty. Detailed descriptions of the girls' beauty (or lack of it) survive for the eighteenth century, for example the case of 13-year-old Caterina Felice Guastuzzi, whom the governors described as not so much beautiful as mediocre in appearance, on account of the shortness of her neck and her protruding shoulders.[48] The conservatory's governors could have been reading from Renaissance treatises on female beauty, which praised long, slender necks and "graceful shoulders," as Parmigianino depicted in his painting, *Madonna of the Long Neck*.[49]

Unlike the Convertite, which sought to save women who had already fallen into a life of vice and disease, the Zitelle made its mission to protect Venice's beautiful young girls before they ever reached that fate. The Zitelle's founders were aware that, as at the Convertite, these beautiful young girls could provide a temptation to those placed in charge of them. Once inside the institution, girls came under the care of a female hierarchy who taught the girls to read and to master a particular skill which would eventually make them suitable marriage partners or, if they chose, nuns in a cloistered convent.[50] Only virgins were allowed to enter the institution, where they were supposed to spend five or six years prior to marriage or entry into a convent.[51] A multi-layered hierarchy ensured that the girls, as well as their superiors, were well supervised. At the lowest level, the female teachers were elected from among the Zitelle boarders; they were responsible for teaching the girls to read, to learn specific skills such as embroidery, and to make sure they prayed and dressed modestly. At the highest level, noblewomen and noblemen filled the roles of *protettrici* and *protettori* who performed the roles of trustees. Day-to-day contact with their girls was restricted to the female hierarchy; even physicians could not visit one of the girls alone, but had to be accompanied by a female administrator (confessors, however, were exempt from this requirement).[52]

Contagion and beautiful females

Isolating these beautiful women was part of Venice's strategy to protect the city's health, defined broadly in moral and physical terms. By placing the Convertite and the Zitelle on the islands of the Giudecca, Venetians ensured that the institutions' inhabitants were physically removed from the mainstream of Venetian life. Cost played an important role in influencing decisions to locate these institutions on islands outside central Venice, but it was not the only factor. Cultural anxieties about physical and moral pollution have often been intertwined with anxieties about disease and danger.[53] Physical isolation lessened the chances of contagion, a complex concept in early modern Europe in which material and metaphoric understandings of the process of contagion overlapped.[54] For example, it was argued that the act of reading romances could induce lovesickness in vulnerable women, because contagion could act at a distance, through sight or the imagination.[55] Church authorities repeatedly referred to heresy as a contagious disease; Pope Paul III had even complained to the Venetian ambassador that heresy had reached epidemic levels in Venice and therefore posed a threat of contagion to the rest of Italy.[56]

Touch was another more direct method of transmission. Touch (or *tangere*) is the root of the word contagion, and hence the focal point of anxieties about and representations of contagion. During the Renaissance, artists represented touch in association with the erotic (sensual pleasure) but also with the dangers of the French disease.[57]

Although theoretically all human bodies were capable of transmitting disease, in practice certain kinds of bodies—women's bodies and Jewish bodies, to name two examples—provoked more anxieties than others. Contemporary art frequently depicted the encounter between Mary Magdalene and the newly risen Christ, often including Jesus' request to Mary Magdalene, *"Noli me tangere"* (Do not touch me).[58] It was the sensuous Mary Magdalene, patron saint of the Convertite, whose touch could potentially pollute Christ before his ascension to heaven. Significantly, Venice's Convertite contained two paintings representing the *Noli me tangere* scene: one painted by Luigi Benfatto, the other by Alvise del Friso, in addition to Palma Giovane's painting on the church's ceiling of the Magdalene being lifted by angels.[59] Venetians enacted these anxieties about sensuous women's polluting touch by restricting their access to sacred space. For example, Venetian law tried to maintain a strict segregation between *meretrici* and respectable women by insisting that disreputable women not attend mass at certain hours and not speak to respectable women.[60] Venetian authorities also tried to protect Venice's secular spaces from these women's "touch." The health department warned that *meretrici* could bring a variety of diseases, including plague. City health authorities specifically targeted immigrant *meretrici*; in 1539, for example, *meretrici* of "foreign origin" (usually from different Italian city-states) were ordered to leave the city on account of the "disorder" they brought, and therefore the risk of plague.[61]

With the establishment of the Convertite in a hidden corner on the island of the Giudecca, Venice's own *meretrici* were removed from the city center, a safe distance from their potentially polluting touch or sight (Figures 4.1 and 4.2). The Zitelle's vulnerable girls were also located on the island of the Giudecca, but clearly visible from the Piazzetta San Marco and the southern part of the city. The decision to locate the institutions of the Zitelle and the Convertite on the islands of the Giudecca marked a shift in Venetian practice from the tradition of integrating charitable institutions into the fabric of neighborhood life to the isolation and removal of these institutions to the outskirts of Venice, a safe distance from the political, symbolic, and residential centers of Venice.[62] Administratively, the Giudecca was part of the city of Venice. In the imagination of city inhabitants, however, the Giudecca was nonetheless regarded as separate and distinct from Venice itself. The sense of separateness derived from its history as well as its location, having served since the tenth century as a refuge for groups of Jews, exiled Venetians, and Eastern Orthodox communities.[63]

One response to the dangers of contagion was physical isolation or quarantine. First instituted in response to the plague in 1377 in Ragusa (modern day Dubrovnik, Croatia), quarantine became a regular practice throughout central and northern Italian city-states during the fifteenth century, beginning with removal of the sick to isolation hospitals and banning of transport of people and goods to and from a city's walls or jurisdiction. Venice first imposed quarantine in 1423. By the mid-sixteenth century, Venice's health board (the *Sanità*) routinely isolated

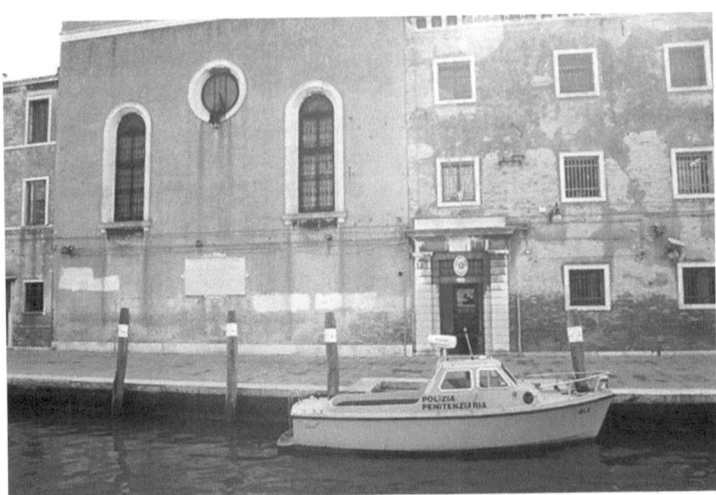

Figure 4.1   Photo of the *Convertite* taken in 2002. The convent has been converted into a women's prison

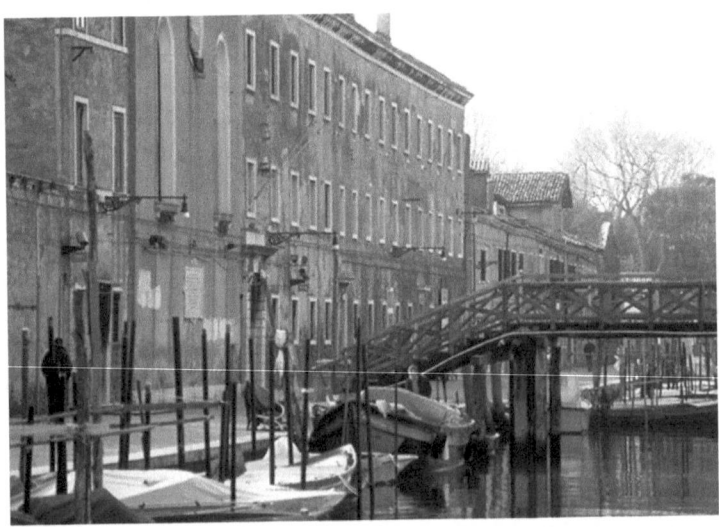

Figure 4.2   Side view of the bridge leading to the *Convertite*. Photo taken in 2002

the sick and the potentially infected on islands, the Lazzaretto Vecchio and Nuovo.[64] This practice coincided with the removal and isolation of *meretrici* from the Incurables hospital to the Convertite on the island of Giudecca, a related practice which suggests how social, moral, and physical ideas of contagion may have informed the sixteenth-century practice of quarantine. Quarantine can be interpreted too narrowly as a purely medical practice in Renaissance Italy, when in fact it formed part of a wider response of expulsion or isolation of people (especially foreigners, prostitutes, and Jews) regarded as dangerous to a city's spiritual and physical health.[65] It was during the early sixteenth century, for example, that Venice's Jewish ghetto was first physically segregated and isolated, another practice of "quarantine" applied to a marginalized people, suspected of contagion both moral and physical. If they survived, however, plague victims endured only temporary physical and social isolation, while Jews and repentant *meretrici* faced permanent physical isolation and enclosure at opposite ends of Venice. Social control was therefore one technique to prevent the spread of contagion.

Financial and other difficulties: Weakening commitment to French disease control

The financial realties of running an institution created difficulties that ultimately eroded the female asylums' ability to provide refuge for women who had contracted or who were likely to contract the French disease. In order to solve financial problems, the female asylums relied more and more on the support of Venice's artisan and merchant classes, who were more interested in the benefits these institutions could offer to their families, such as the education of girls, than in disease control. By the seventeenth century, the Convertite's inhabitants were typically either noblemen's former lovers or concubines, not women with multiple sexual partners, or virgins who could not afford to enter a traditional convent.

Initially, Venice's Convertite supported itself through the nuns' labor: they ran a printing press which produced religious titles such as editions of Peter Lombard's *Sentences*, and they spun thread sufficiently well to undersell the city's established putting-out system of home labor.[66] When the convent was founded, no one could have anticipated the devastating impact that church reform would have on the financial survival of female monastic institutions. During the last session of the church's Council of Trent (1545–63), reformers imposed strict cloister (enclosure) on all female religious institutions, which meant that any type of physical contact between female religious and the outside world was forbidden. Specifically, female religious could no longer leave convents in order to teach or to nurse the sick, nor could they engage in economic activities that required physical contact with the outside world, such as spinning, printing, and baking. Strict cloister unintentionally imposed significant hardships on convents throughout Europe; ultimately, convents covered these costs by raising the minimum spiritual dowry that each nun was required to bring on entering a convent. It became increasingly difficult for women from modest financial backgrounds to become nuns after the Council of Trent's reforms.[67]

Venice's Convertite could no longer run its printing press or spin thread, placing the convent in immediate and protracted financial distress. After the embarrassing sexual scandal involving the convent's first rector, the Venetian government intervened in 1564 to assist the institution by requiring that a certain percentage of fines imposed on criminals be sent to the Convertite.[68] The convent nonetheless continued to struggle financially. During the lean years of crop failure and widespread hunger that marked the 1590s, for example, more than 350 nuns and 150 chickens, whose screeches constantly interrupted the choir nuns at prayer, crowded into the Convertite's sadly inadequate buildings. One of the four dormitories lacked an intact ceiling and failed to protect the nuns from cold in winter and heat in summer, the cells were divided makeshift-style with canvas rather than wood, and two of the church's altars failed to meet the minimum requirements for celebration of the Mass, since they were constructed of wood rather than stone. The nuns also suffered from hunger.[69] Conditions improved after the 1590s, although the Convertite was never wealthy. Nonetheless, by the seventeenth century, the Convertite provided shelter, food, and a modest standard of living, an improvement, to be sure, for Venice's desperate poor.

The Convertite struggled to fill its ranks only with "fallen women." In fact, less than one-half of the women who entered the Convertite in the mid-seventeenth century fulfilled the minimum requirements for entry, that is, being *meretrici* or women who had lost their virginity outside of marriage. Fifty women, or 48 percent, either came directly from a different institution, the Casa del Soccorso, or were listed as having been "raised from the devil's jaws," the euphemism for having lost one's virginity outside of marriage.[70]

It is, unfortunately, not possible to reconstruct the life histories of all or even the majority of the women who willingly took vows at the Convertite. But a limited composite portrait is possible based on surviving demographic data for the mid-seventeenth century, in which names and ages were recorded. For the years 1656 to 1675, the convent's records of who entered survive; during these 20 years, a total of 104 women entered the Convertite.[71] Young women (ages 15–24) accounted for the majority of women who took vows at the Convertite. The Convertite did not serve as a retirement home for aging prostitutes, as its founders feared.[72] The vast majority of women who entered the convent were young and still capable of years of sexual activity. Of the 104 women entering between 1656 and 1675, 20 (19 percent) were between the ages of 15 and 19, and 43 (41 percent) were between the ages of 20 and 24. Fully 60 percent of the new nuns were therefore between the ages of 15 and 24.[73]

A few young women and girls entered the Convertite because they had been victims of rape. Rape victims were few in number in the convent, but they provide the most dramatic—and sympathetic—examples of rebellion. What undermined the convent's ability to provide a permanent home for victims of sexual violence was its uniform emphasis on repentance for all its residents, regardless of whether the woman who entered was a former prostitute, concubine, estranged wife, or rape victim. By failing to make distinctions between these different types of sexual experiences, the convent's governors inadvertently sparked rebellion and discontent. Fourteen-year-old Agnesina, for example, had been living with her mother when she was raped in 1592. Explaining that her mother led a "bad life" and hence was at least partially responsible for her daughter's misfortune, relatives brought Agnesina to the Convertite, saying that they did not know how to save her "on account of her poverty." What her relatives regarded as an act of mercy apparently seemed like an act of punishment to young Agnesina: exactly nine months after taking religious vows, on the same day and at the very same hour, she and two others nuns set fire to one of the buildings. Because of this crime, she was imprisoned for eight years in the convent's internal prison, until she and her accomplices broke free and escaped one night, fleeing to relatives' homes where they remained hidden. Life outside the convent disappointed her, however, for reasons unexplained in the surviving sources. In July of 1600, shortly after her dramatic escape, she petitioned to be allowed to return the convent. As the Venetian patriarch explained in his supplication to the authorities in Rome, "with great remorse of her conscience, she would willingly return to the monastery, but no longer in the prison." She was granted her wish.[74]

Since rape (especially gang rape) was one of the principal ways in which teenage girls were forced into prostitution throughout Europe during this period, convent authorities may have thought they were fulfilling the founders' intentions by allowing rape victims to enter.[75] They were presumably preventing these girls from a life of prostitution. But the convent's hierarchy, including a female abbess and a male confessor, was ill prepared to meet the emotional and psychological needs of these girls and women. One rape victim threatened suicide at the Convertite in the mainland city of Padua. A noblewoman and nun at the prestigious Benedictine convent of San Michele in Este, Sister Gabriele Roverani was subject to a violent rape inside the convent walls. Moved from the city of Este to the city of Padua, Sister Gabriele believed that she was going to be moved to another Benedictine convent. Instead, she was placed in the Convertite, neither Benedictine nor full of virgins, as she herself had been until her rape. Upon discovering the truth about her new home, she "burst out in most devout cries exclaiming of having been betrayed." She was inconsolable because of the offense done to her reputation, and that of her relatives. After her superiors and even Cardinal Barbarigo tried to placate her to no avail, they finally wrote to the authorities at the Vatican on her behalf, claiming that they feared for her life, and for her soul should she take her life. Her story must have finally touched a nerve at the Vatican, since, after four long years of appeals, she was finally allowed to enter a Benedictine convent.[76] Sister Gabriele was hardly a likely candidate for prostitution, even after her rape. The decision to send her to the Convertite indicates more of a desire to protect the honor of the Benedictine convents than to prevent a woman from becoming a prostitute. By placing her in a place of "penitence," ecclesiastical authorities sabotaged her morale and undermined the significance of the meaning of repentance. These dramatic stories of rebellion were hardly typical, since rape victims always constituted a minority of the convent's residents.[77]

More common were the former lovers of prominent Venetian men. Although the Convertite did not serve as a retirement home for nobleman's aged former lovers, it nevertheless did provide a home for former lovers who were still young. It is unclear from the evidence in these cases why the woman entered the convent: perhaps her former lover had been pressured to marry a woman of the same social class. Noblemen willing to pay their former lover's expenses probably did so for only one woman: a casual sexual relationship was unlikely to inspire this degree of loyalty. It is possible that these relationships were monogamous, or at least serially monogamous, and hence not necessarily the most effective target for the prevention of the spread of the French disease.

The case of Sister Maria Lion provides an example of the enduring ties, even in the absence of sexual relations, between noblemen and their lovers. On October 7, 1626, the nobleman Tomà Lion paid one of his frequent visits to his former lover, now called Sister Maria Lion, at the Convertite. She had entered the Convertite only weeks earlier and made all outwards signs of conversion. She claimed that she was converted, repented her past errors, submitted to having her hair cut, wore the monastic habit, and changed her name, in accordance with the custom whereby a nun abandons her worldly name and assumes a new identity. But the name she chose was significant: she adopted her lover's last name, a name that clearly indicated her affiliation with the noble Lion family. Tomà Lion paid her expenses at the Convertite. He brought his friends along when he visited the convent and saw her only at the convent's parlor, where the nuns were kept physically separated from visitors by iron grating. No sexual improprieties were mentioned, nor love letters: The visits were about sociability, not sexuality. Since the Council of Trent's regulations explicitly forbade even sociable visits to nuns from laypeople without a special license (which would not have been given to a former lover, in all probability), Tomà was in breech of the law. On December 21, the Convertite's governors assured the secular authorities responsible for convents (the *Provveditori sopra Monasteri*) that Lion had ceased visiting his former lover. The authorities dismissed him without further punishment and required only that he not see her again.[78] Given that the convent did not keep systematic records of who paid expenses, this story is suggestive, rather than conclusive. Nonetheless, this case is not the only evidence that former lovers paid convent expenses and tried to maintain contact.[79]

For some former concubines of noblemen, however, a life of permanent penitence was an unattractive option, so they rebelled and fled. In 1618, for example, one of the nuns successfully escaped from the Convertite, after months of complaining that she wanted to leave. She manifested her discontent by refusing to comply with the rules: she grew her hair long, wore curls, and clothed herself in whatever worldly clothes she could find.[80] In doing so, she was attempting to regain beauty, defined by long hair and fashionable clothing, which she had been required to sacrifice within the convent. Cutting a woman's hair was an important part of the ritual process of becoming a nun, dramatically illustrating the rejection of worldly vices such as vanity. But for some nuns their physical transformation was only temporary, as they both overtly and covertly violated rules regarding modest dress. When the Patriarch (Venice's equivalent of an archbishop) formally visited the Convertite in 1625, he criticized the nuns' attention to their own physical beauty. Some wore their hair long, uncovered, and donned gold jewelry, while others more subtly broke rules by wearing silk veils and silk underclothing.[81]

This particular escaped nun's discontent had manifested itself in a variety of acts beyond disobedience regarding hair and clothing. She even threatened to set the convent on fire if she were not permitted to leave. As she explained to Sister Felice prior to her escape, she rejected not only monastic life and all of its discipline, but also the very idea of perpetual penitence on which the convent was founded. "This is not my place, I was put here for safety, I have finished my penitence and I want to go away," she told Sister Felice.[82] This nun's comments—as well as the detailed case described below—illustrate the difficulties that the Convertite and other female asylums encountered in trying to fulfill their mandate.

Case study of a rebellious nun: Angela Giustiniana

The case of Angela Giustiniana, well-documented because she stood trial before the Holy Office, is particularly instructive in illustrating the limitations of the convent's appeal to "fallen women." Prior to entering the Convertite, Angela Giustiniana had been abandoned by her long-standing boyfriend, Leonardo Marcello, a nobleman. The relationship had endured some six or seven years before its demise during the winter months of 1624. The couple quarreled frequently, according to Angela, and then Leonardo stopped visiting her at all. After two months' absence, Angela grew desperate. "I was very tormented," she explained to the Inquisitors at the Holy Office, "and it came to my mind a woman named Annetta Zonfina who stayed in Canareggio who knew a remedy to make men return."[83] With a bit of Leonardo's urine in her possession, Annetta would be able to perform several rituals to ensure his return to Angela.

Before Annetta's remedies had a chance to work, however, Angela became sick, with which disease or symptoms she did not say. She sought refuge in the Convertite, where she stayed 18 months, during which time she returned to good health. But she remained devoted to the task that had occupied her attention outside the convent: trying to get Leonardo Marcello to return to her. In the midst of orthodox Catholic life, Angela practiced sorcery—at first on the sly, but gradually growing bolder. One witness claimed that she had bragged about her powers to other nuns: she claimed that she could make men return at will or make them die. She earned the enmity of one woman, Sister Giacinta, who complained of her "dirty and evil tongue."[84]

In her defense, Angela explained that she had practiced sorcery only once inside the convent; any statements suggesting that she had regularly practiced sorcery were false accusations from her enemies. "I disgusted them," she explained to the Holy Office. "I was crying, and

I wanted to leave, and I made them furious ... They invented this falsity (about practicing sorcery) because they were afraid that I would ask for the dowry of 200 ducats which I had left them."[85] Like all convents, the Convertite required a dowry from women who entered in order to cover costs. The 200-ducat dowry was modest by the standards of other Venetian convents, but nonetheless represented a significant outlay for people of modest incomes.

After having left the Convertite, Angela was free to pursue her sorcery without interference from hostile nuns. At age 34, she wondered if she, like Camilla Savioni from Chapter 3, still possessed enough physical attractiveness to keep Leonardo interested and used magic in an effort to bind his affections to her.[86] But Leonardo Marcello himself brought a halt to her fervent activities when he denounced her to the Holy Office: Perhaps he feared that Angela's magic could be efficacious and harm him. Or perhaps he was simply tired of her efforts to win him back. Although it is not possible to identify Leonardo Marcello beyond a shadow of doubt, since the Marcellos were a large family with many branches, there was a Leonardo Marcello who wrote his last will and testament in 1626, the very same year that Angela was denounced to the Holy Office. If these men were one and the same (which is probable), then Leonardo denounced his former lover just one month prior to writing his last will in which he left virtually all of his rather small fortune to his wife, also named Angela, and made no mention of a lover, nor of any children.[87] He would have been 41 years old in 1626.[88] Leonardo may have been trying to end the love affair peaceably first by placing Angela Giustiniana in the Convertite with a 200-ducat dowry; when that strategy failed, he resorted to the Holy Office.

Whatever his motive, Angela's reaction was clear: she preferred life outside the convent. The Convertite's failure to "convert" Angela to its religious and theological program illustrates its limitations as an institution on at least three levels. First, Angela never regarded her problems as being the result of her own moral failings. As she defined it, her problem was practical: her lover had left her and she wanted him back. For an institution to be effective, it must make some effort to address its clients' needs on their terms. Of course the Convertite, a Catholic convent, would not have aided Angela in her effort to win back Leonardo Marcello. But it could have provided a richer framework for her to understand her own problems: Biblical stories of human betrayal and abandonment, of solace found in trusting God's love rather than human love, may have resonated more with Angela's experience than the story of Mary Magdalene the penitent. The Convertite's narrow response to women's problems, and its single solution—penitence—for one and all, thereby undercut its effectiveness in converting women like Angela to a life within its walls.

Next, the Convertite did not meet Angela's expectations for the kind of community in which she could live. She did not build enduring friendships, win anyone's approval, nor even manage to get along with the other nuns. Angela's personal difficulties within the institution suggest a gulf between the convent's culture and the culture with which Angela was familiar. The gulf between the life of a concubine and the life of a nun, even a "converted nun," was too wide for Angela to bridge.

Finally, the convent's priests and abbess did not effectively explain the difference between orthodox Catholic belief and magic to the new entrants to the convent. Angela blended references to Catholic saints with magical practices and borrowed from Catholic rituals when trying to secure Leonardo's love. She recognized no difference between these two systems of belief and practice.

> One time I said 13 Our Fathers and the penitentials to Saint Anthony while kneeling ... and then this prayer, in which (it was) my intention that Saint Anthony inspire in the heart of Signor Lunardo (Leonardo) Marcello with whom I was so enamored, that he return to me to make peace, because we used to fight often. And I said these prayers for 13 or more days, and I held a candle lit in (my) hand, and a figure of Saint Anthony.[89]

Her understanding of religion was instrumental: prayer would help her achieve her goals. The primary appeal of the convent was to women who clearly wished to become permanent nuns, but unfortunately they had nothing to repent. The virgins who entered the convent during the seventeenth century signaled the institution's failure to fulfill its mandate as part of Venice's response ot the French disease and effort to secure places of refuge for "fallen women."

The virginity scandal

Only in a convent for fallen women would the presence of virgins cause a scandal. In 1621, several of the oldest nuns in the Convertite denounced the prioress for admitting virgins into the convent under the pretext of paying debts. These young virgins, they wrote, were destroying the convent's calm atmosphere, since the prioress failed to discipline them and they danced, roamed freely, and made a racket in the dormitories and refectory. The nuns denounced the prioress with the strongest possible language: under her rule, the convent was becoming more of a "bordello than a sanctuary" and that "at the Tower of Babel one did not find such confusion as one finds continuously in our choir, dormitories and refectory."[90] It was an odd image: the presence of virgins in the convent created the atmosphere of a bordello. This apparent paradox would have seemed like perfectly sensible imagery to early modern Venetians, since bordellos were associated with chaos and the lack of rules.

The presence of virgins in the Convertite violated the convent's rules, established in order "to raise souls from the stench of sin, to liberate them from the slavery of the devil, and to put them in a place of security."[91] Admitting virgins therefore amounted to a relaxation of the regulations—a symptom of disorder, not of monastic discipline. Because of the convent's unique mission, the older nuns could simultaneously condemn the prioress for admitting virgins and for running a bordello-like convent: Both signaled a breakdown in order and discipline. The older nuns referred to the prioress as a *meretrice*, in this context clearly a figure of speech to condemn her venality rather than her sexual behavior. The use of the word *meretrice* in this context shows how this word was often used to denote disorder or lack of discipline, not literally prostitution. Furthermore, critics accused the prioress of being "more stone and wood than human creature, the cause of so many relaxations [of rules] and scandals."[92] In 1632, in response to repeated denunciations, the Venetian Senate condemned the convent for admitting virgins as an abuse and blamed its financial problems on the ever-increasing number of nuns.[93]

Financial struggles were at the root of the prioress's decision to admit virgins. As mentioned previously, ever since the Convertite became a cloistered convent in 1563, the convent struggled to survive. To stabilize its finances, the Senate voted in 1564 to give the Convertite a certain fixed percentage of all fines imposed on criminals. In 1622, the Senate became even more specific: *meretrici* should be taxed in order to support the institution that advocated their conversion from sin. Each parish priest was encouraged to identify public prostitutes, some of whom allegedly lived comfortably and paid rents of more than 40 ducats.[94] The Senate's decision appealed to the desire to make the punishment fit the crime: *meretrici* should pay for their sins by helping their sisters turn to God.

Unfortunately for the Convertite, the wages of sin were difficult to collect and never provided reliable income. The Senate had to remind the magistrates responsible for disbursing funds to the convent to ful-fill their duties in 1628.[95] But two years later the problem resurfaced: the convent's money had been usurped, according to an anonymous informant.[96] Complaints continued as the years passed: in 1646, the Convertite's governors claimed that the Republic of Venice owed them a whopping sum: a total of 3086 ducats, 7 grossi.[97] The state may have retained the convent's share of criminal fines in order to finance its war against Turkey, which also started in 1646. On April 6, 1646, the Senate informed the governors of the Convertite that the institution, because it was dedicated to God, had a particular obligation to support this war, a religious war against the Infidel.[98]

Far more lucrative than taxation of sin were the large spiritual dow-ries that virgins brought with them to enter the Convertite. Although the sources on the amount of each woman's spiritual dowry assets are incomplete, the records that do survive suggest that virgins consist-ently paid more than fallen women to enter the convent. Seventeen-year-old Menega, a virgin, brought 450 ducats as her spiritual dowry in 1656, whereas the "fallen women" Anzola and Elena, ages 21 and 22 respectively, each brought only 200 ducats as their spiritual dowries.[99] This trend whereby virgins brought twice as much in financial assets as non-virgins apparently started early in the convent's history: the oldest surviving records of convent entrants, dating from 1602 to 1608, show a similar discrepancy in financial assets between virgins and non-virgins. The virgin Medea, recommended for entrance by one of the convent's governors, Bortolamio dal Calice, brought a whopping 350 ducat-dowry in 1602, while Chiaretta, a sailor's daughter with two children of her own, brought a mere 50 ducats in January 1603 and the promise of another 50 ducats in the future. Chiaretta's children also entered the convent, with promises that they would not disturb the other nuns.[100]

Although the practice of admitting virgins into the convent violated the rules, it did ease the convent's chronic financial problems which neither the church nor the state had done much to resolve. During the lean years of the 1590s, the prioress, Sister Clementia, described the urgent needs of the nuns: "At present in our monastery we do not have even the dust of flour, nor bread, nor wine, nor oil, nor any-thing that could sustain us."[101] The church's response—specifically the Venetian Patriarch's response—was to encourage tighter management of the convent's resources. In his 1599 recommendations, the Patriarch demanded a more thorough system of security for the convent's bank. The prioress could not accept monetary gifts by herself, but only in the presence of at least three others: her female deputy (*vicaria*), the scribe, and one of the four treasurers. The treasurers' office should be rotated sufficiently frequently to prevent corruption, according to the Patriarch. Two treasurers would serve for one month, followed the next month by the other two, each opening the convent's bank only in the presence of the other.[102] The Patriarch seemed to regard the convent's fiscal woes solely as a result of theft and mismanagement, not inadequate resources. Little wonder that the prioress and the convent's governors looked for new sources of income in the form of virgins, since cloister prevented the nuns from earning it, while church and state failed to provide adequately for the convent's needs.

But what motivated virgins to enter a convent for repentant *meretrici*? The reason was a strong spiritual vocation, but inadequate funds to enter a convent for virgins. In 1601, for example, Livia Citaredi of Urbino requested admission to the Convertite in the same city, asking for special dispensation since she was a virgin and had never led a dissolute life. As her local bishop explained, "She is so desirous to be a religious that she is content to enter into the monastery of the Convertite of said place [Urbino] where since she is so virtuous the nuns consent to receive her with that dowry she has." The Sacra Congregatione at the Vatican refused permission for her to enter.[103] Fifty years later, 15-year-old Catterina Santi Bononi, a virgin from Bologna, received the same answer when she requested entrance to her city's Convertite, "for her poverty she cannot serve the Lord God in another monastery."[104]

The spiraling costs of monastic life after the Council of Trent prevented ordinary pious women from becoming nuns. While rich families dumped their daughters into convents to preserve the family fortune from the even greater costs of marriage dowries, genuinely pious women found themselves with fewer options to pursue religious life than their predecessors in the early sixteenth century. Safely enclosed behind the walls of the convent, nuns spared the church the embarrassment of sexual scandal, but were unable to support themselves. Pious women with no other options for a religious life willingly entered convents for fallen women, thereby providing the necessary revenue to keep the institutions running.

The surviving entry records for the years 1602–8 and 1656–75 provide supporting evidence that the Convertite attracted ordinary pious women of the merchant and artisan classes. Although entering nun's father's occupation was recorded for only 9 of the 28 women from the earlier group and for 21 of the 104 women from the later group, one place of work remained constant: the Arsenal.[105] The Arsenal was Venice's enormous shipbuilding factory covering approximately

60 acres in the sestiere of Castello; as Europe's largest factory during the sixteenth century, the Arsenal employed about 10 percent of Venice's workers, including reasonably well-paid craftsmen, such as shipwrights and caulkers (among the occupations listed for fathers of women entering the Convertite). Marriage dowries for daughters of master craftsmen ranged from 200 to 400 ducats during the mid-seventeenth century,[106] precisely the same range as spiritual dowries for the Convertite but only about one-tenth the cost of spiritual dowries for Venice's traditional convents.[107]

Despite concern that *meretrici*, even repentant *meretrici*, would corrupt virgins, the two groups managed to coexist. In Tuscany in 1579, the convent's statutes explicitly stated that virgins not be allowed to enter the convent for their own protection: "We're not meant for everyone, but for those who've fallen into trouble. Yet not even for this reason should we accept virgins—even when their expenses will be paid and they come with convertite who are their mothers—because of the danger they'd be putting themselves in by being exposed to the conversation of the convertite."[108] In practice, however, these convents admitted virgins without official permission throughout the Italian peninsula. In Ferrara, Gubbio, and Naples, the convents had been admitting virgins who wanted to receive an education for decades, claiming that they were unaware that this practice was unacceptable. Once the girls came of age, they were often allowed to take vows, although they were virgins. The prioress of the Naples convent defended the practice on the grounds that these young women lacked family support and had no other options: By admitting them to the convent, she was removing them from "evident danger" and performing a work of "infinite piety."[109]

Virgins did not account for the concentration of young women as new entrants to the Convertite. Both "fallen women" and virgins shared the same age distribution.[110] Despite similarities in age, it may have been difficult to integrate these two groups in one convent. The convent's spatial organization may have helped smooth relations between virgins and "fallen women." The convent had four separate dormitories to house more than 350 women. Tensions flared from time to time, as the denunciations against the presence of virgins indicate, but the convent was large enough to enable groups to form their own friendships and allies. Although the Patriarch protested against the presence of factions within the convent that destroyed the spirit of community, these very factions may have enabled women from startlingly different backgrounds to coexist.[111] Some of the nuns kept puppies and small dogs as pets, formed close friendships with a few of the nuns and nursed bitter resentments against others, and kept their own, private chickens to supplement their diets with the eggs, thereby creating private worlds of friendship and attachment.[112] In addition to virgins and former concubines of noblemen, a third group of women—estranged or battered wives—found temporary refuge within the Convertite and further altered the convent's nature and function.[113] This group proved the most powerful in shaping the institution to meet their own needs, rather than having the institution impose its agenda for reform upon these women.

In this respect, the Convertite resembled other convents of the time, largely filled with women who lacked a spiritual vocation, rebelling against their families' decisions to place them in convents by breaking minor rules such as keeping pets and wearing fine clothing.[114] Nuns were supposed to take their vows voluntarily, but families could nonetheless place them under tremendous pressure to enter convents. Small infractions of rules therefore did not single out the Convertite as an institutional failure, since nuns in traditional convents experienced similar difficulties in obeying the rigorous demands of monastic life. The Convertite was, however, a special convent, designed to transform the lives of fallen women, a need that was seen to be more urgent in the context of the French disease epidemic of the sixteenth century. Because different groups (virgins from respectable families, wives seeking separations, noblemen needing a refuge for their former lovers) successfully adapted the institution to their own needs, the institution no longer fulfilled its original mandate.

The Zitelle: Dowries and education for artisan girls

Similarly, the Zitelle, the asylum designed to prevent beautiful, poor girls from being deflowered and becoming infected with the French disease, also changed over time to fulfill the needs of Venice's artisans. When old enough to marry, each of the girls received a dowry. Beautiful, literate, able to sew, possessing a dowry, these young virgins possessed everything they needed to compete successfully on the marriage market. The overwhelming majority (roughly 85 percent) chose to marry rather than enter a convent; their husbands came from solid artisan backgrounds, working as spice vendors, masons, weavers, tailors, servants, and so forth. Their desirability as brides made their status somewhat enviable among struggling artisan families. By the seventeenth century, the girls in the Zitelle no longer came from the ranks of Venice's poor and marginal, but

from the "deserving poor," that is, from artisan families who were struggling to make ends meet.[115] Venice's Zitelle was not alone in responding
to pressure to meet the needs of the "respectable poor" rather than the
city's destitute families. In Rome, S. Caterina della Rosa was founded in
the mid-sixteenth century to rescue prostitutes' daughters from following
their mothers' careers. By 1600, however, the institution accepted any
young woman with a mere "hint of danger."[116] The impoverished young
girls, beautiful or not, were left to manage on their own. No doubt some
of them survived through prostitution. Neither the Convertite nor the
Zitelle therefore protected the poorest in Venice from being deflowered
and possibly infected with the French disease.

A New institution, old problems

Although both the Zitelle and the Convertite came to be regarded as
failures by the late seventeenth century, state and ecclesiastical authorities continued to define the French disease as a problem of women's
bodies and women's unregulated sexuality. The solutions they proposed
for these problems were more of the same—a new house of penitence
for fallen women, but one that would specifically benefit the poor. In
1701, a new asylum, somewhat cumbersomely called the Pious Place
for the Poor Penitent Sinners of Saint Job, or more simply the Penitenti,
began accepting penitent *meretrici*. Since the penitent women who
entered did not adopt the religious life, they were not required to
observe strict cloister. Their expenses were therefore lower than the
Convertite's. The cost of entry was only one ducat; the house's expenses
were largely paid through charity.[117] Furthermore, the Penitenti housed
only 36 women, roughly one-tenth the size of the Convertite, which cut
down on operating costs but substantially reduced the Penitenti's social
impact.[118] Significantly, the Penitenti dropped beauty as a requirement
for entrance, signaling a shift in emphasis from beauty to poverty as the
principal cause of prostitution and disease.

What remained the same was the emphasis on women's bodies and
women's need for moral reform. As Kevin Siena has shown in the case
of the eighteenth-century Lock Asylum for the Reception of Penitent
Women in London, cure for women was a two-stage process: first the
body, then the soul. Men underwent only the first stage of this process.[119] Venice's policy was similar. Female patients being treated for
the French disease were transferred directly from the *Incurabili* hospital
to the Penitenti, while male patients were merely released from the
hospital. On October 31, 1793, for example, the physician-in-charge

noted that five women were "completely cured" and ready to go the following day to the Penitenti. Between 1793 and 1795, the hospital for the *Incurabili* treated and "cured" between 116 and 137 French disease patients each year, fairly equally divided between men and women. When space was available, former female patients were sent to the Penitenti, but men were free to go where they pleased.[120]

The Penitenti redefined the problem of women's sexuality as the result of poverty rather than beauty. During the early eighteenth century, various Catholic reformers emphasized that poverty, rather than wealth, more often acted as a temptation to sin in people's lives.[121] Throughout Europe, political elites redefined poverty's fundamental causes during the eighteenth century, from what Sandra Cavallo has called the "natural causes" of illness or death of a family member to social causes (unemployment, low wages).[122] Complex, slow changes in the economy, including the development of industries and the decline of seasonal migration to cities in favor of permanent migration, spurred some observers to look for underlying economic changes as the cause of poverty rather than individual sin. Although these ideas became more clearly and systematically expressed in later intellectual movements of the eighteenth century (especially the cameralists who in turn influenced the Enlightenment philosophers), preoccupations with redefining poverty and reforming charity were evident from the beginning of the eighteenth-century.[123]

In Venice, the Penitenti's regulations reflected changing attitudes and provided a critique of the Convertite's practices of admitting women of financial means. The Penitenti stipulated that entrants must be poor, "and so miserable, that they have no means of living without sinning. And therefore are excluded the well-to-do prostitutes, and those that have an honest art for procuring food, and those that have relatives, or pious persons, who could, or would help them, and in sum all those who could in another manner save themselves."[124] Venetians were therefore making distinctions among "fallen women" and no longer grouping them all together in one institution, a trend taking place in other Italian cities as well. As Sandra Cavallo has suggested, this change might be linked to the declining importance of female honor as a fundamental category.[125] Rape victims, separated wives, and former concubines had all experienced risks to their honor, which explained why they were housed together in one institution.[126] With the creation of a new method of categorizing women according to economic status, Venetian authorities thereby reduced the importance of sexual honor as fundamental to women's experience. It is probably not possible to disentangle the web of influences that brought about this change, since the elites were no doubt not simply imposing change but also responding to it and in turn perpetuating long-term changes in social attitudes. Although Venetian authorities had shifted their emphasis from beauty to poverty, they nonetheless still focused on the dangers of the female body.

Contemporary medical theory regarding the risks of beauty had changed as well. For example, in 1718 the physician Carlo Musitano criticized the theory that the French disease had arisen within the body of a single woman who had experienced an unusual amount of sexual intercourse with many different men. "But it is false," he argued, "that semen putrefies through excessive use of Venus." Human beings had made "immoderate use of Venus ever since the World was created, and especially after the fecund benediction: 'Increase and multiply, fill the earth.'"[127] Furthermore, beautiful women alone were not responsible for the disease's transmission, but "both beautiful and ugly" prostitutes who sexual relations with the French army after the French invasion and retreat of the late fifteenth century.[128] Nonetheless, eighteenth-century theories still focused primarily on women's bodies, with the idea still circulating in France that the mixture of different men's semen in a woman's body could produce ulcers, putrefaction, and ultimately was responsible for the spread of disease.[129] Creative entrepreneurs meanwhile sold such dubious items as "chocolate aphrodisiacs" that simultaneously supposedly cured disease: seduction, pleasure, and medicine were all linked in this one product.[130] Men could pursue their pleasures, but women's bodies were still treated as a threat to public health, best enclosed, at least temporarily, in institutions.

The link between the Penitenti and the hospital for the Incurables became much stronger than the link between the hospital and the Convertite had been. Once "cured," women were often released directly from the hospital to the Penitenti. A clean bill of health, signed by a doctor, was required for entry into the Penitenti, on the grounds that a sick woman was not in immediate danger of committing any sin. This rule about only admitting healthy women proved difficult to follow since many women who had allegedly been cured of the French disease fell sick again later. The governors of the Penitenti repeatedly lamented that the house was in danger of becoming a hospital, since so many women were sick from the French disease. The governors emphasized that only healthy women could be accepted and that those who fell sick would be returned to the hospital for Incurables, but it was apparently difficult in practice to enforce the rule about admitting only healthy women.[131] If the disease they suffered from was what we know as modern venereal syphilis, then it would not be surprising that apparently "cured" women suffered from later relapses. For contemporary authorities, relapse was regarded as the result of the difficulty of treating particular cases of the French disease. Female patients who acquired disease through prostitution could appear to be well externally, but in fact still had the disease internally.[132] Treatment of these cases therefore required close collaboration with medical authorities.

Other rules besides the ones regarding illness were difficult to enforce as well, especially the one regarding the minimum age for entry. In 1730, the governors established the minimum age for entrance as 12 years old, even though much younger girls were "deflowered and ruined."[133] The governors were probably reacting to the case of Teresa Veneranda Bortoluci, the eight-year-old daughter of a weaver and his wife Anzola. After having been deflowered (the name of her rapist was not recorded in the Penitenti's records) and infected with the French disease, she spent a long period in the hospital for the Incurables, before moving to the Penitenti in 1730.[134] Such a heart-wrenching case may have caused the governors to suspend their rule against under-age applicants, only to have the rule restated at a subsequent meeting.

Teresa Bortoluci was not the only case of a young child having been raped and infected with the French disease. In 1793, six-year-old Lucia Florissa apparently contracted the French disease from a 29-year-old man who rented the same bed in a small apartment in Venice. This case illustrates the problems that many working-class parents faced in trying to protect their daughters. Lucia's parents, Iseppo and Domenica, immigrants from neighboring Istria, could not live with their daughter, because he was a sailor and she worked as a domestic servant. Lucia's mother, Domenica, arranged for her to stay in Venice with a woman named Cattarina who came from the same town in Istria.[135]

Because this case involved a six-year-old, the authorities in charge investigated the sleeping arrangements thoroughly. Seven people all slept in the same room on three different beds: a married couple who shared one bed, the father of the wife had a bed to himself, and finally the third bed was rented to non-kin boarders, including Cattarina, her daughter, six-year-old Lucia, and 29-year-old Domenico De Silvestro, a basket-maker from Friuli who had lived in Venice for nine months. Interviews with the married couple revealed that Domenico did have the opportunity to have sexual relations with Lucia, since she went to bed first, followed by Domenico; only later did the others follow. Lucia's mother discovered what had happened when she came to visit her daughter, who cried in pain when she tried to urinate. The girl was eventually taken to the hospital of the Incurabili, where the examining doctor diagnosed her with the French disease. No signs of disease were evident on Domenico's body. Nonetheless, he was found guilty by the *Esecutori contra la Bestemmia* and sentenced to three years' galley labor, no doubt because of the girl's extreme youth.[136] Lucia's mother requested that Lucia be discharged from the hospital to the orphanage of the Pietà, close to where she lived so visits would be possible.[137] The authorities believed that poverty made young girls and women vulnerable to sexual exploitation and therefore to disease, but their solution required that young girls be removed from their parents' care. Parents were held responsible for inadequately protecting their child and punished with the forced removal of their child. Although Venice's working classes struggled to find adequate housing for their families, Venetian authorities chose to place children in institutions rather than provide means of helping entire families.

For adult women, however, the Penitenti did serve as a means of social rehabilitation, enabling former *meretrici* to re-enter Venetian society in new roles. Physically and symbolically, the Penitenti played a very different role from that of the Convertite, tucked out-of-site on the island of the Giudecca. Located on the outskirts of the working-class neighborhood of Cannaregio, the female inhabitants of the Penitenti were not permanently isolated from the residential life of Venice proper. On the northern side of the city, closest to the mainland, Cannaregio was a transitional neighborhood where newcomers to Venice often lived.[138] Instead of isolating these women on a separate island, the Penitenti occupied space within the heart of Venice's struggling neighborhoods. Between 1701 and 1731, the majority of women who entered the Penitenti came from Cannaregio; the neighborhood which contributed the second largest number of women was, unsurprisingly, working-class Castello, with its large population of Arsenal workers and recent Greek immigrants.[139]

Women who entered the Penitenti were not required to stay permanently. They could leave in order to marry, enter a convent, or go into domestic service, as long as the governors of the Penitenti approved of the potential husband or employer. Success within the institution made domestic service a possibility for these women, who had trouble finding employers willing to trust them. But domestic service brought potential dangers, as the governors of the institution knew all too well: an unscrupulous employer could seduce his servant.[140] Ironically, women who emerged from the Penitenti faced many of the same economic and social constraints that women two centuries earlier had faced: limited economic opportunities, restrictions against women joining guilds, and the possibility of a career in domestic service, bringing restricted earnings and sexual politics within the household. Female asylums, whether in their sixteenth- or eighteenth-century form, did not tackle the social, economic, and cultural conditions which had made Venetian women vulnerable to exposure to the French disease.

The ongoing problems associated with the French disease—the increased number of beggars, too sick to work; the vulnerability of young girls to either seduction or rape—inspired a host of institutional responses during the sixteenth century, from the hospital for Incurables to the various female asylums, including the Convertite, the Zitelle, and the Penitenti. Institutional health care in Venice was organized according to type of disease, with different hospitals for those suffering from acute, infectious diseases, and for those suffering from chronic, endemic diseases, such as the French disease. The type of care for French disease patients also varied according to gender, with men having greater access to hospitals and women being pressured to enter asylums that removed them from society until adulthood (in the case of girls) or for the rest of their lives. The female asylums were founded for a dual purpose: to protect the rest of society from the danger these beautiful females posed as both moral and biological contagions, as well as to protect, provide shelter, and improve the lives of these women and girls.

When the Penitenti was established during the eighteenth century with strong links to the Incurables hospital and a focus on poverty rather than beauty, the French disease became a continuing problem for the institution. Although women were supposed to be treated and cured prior to admission, relapse often occurred. For the governors of the Penitenti, the problem of relapse never led them to question the efficacy of French disease treatment themselves. Instead, they lamented the difficulty presented in knowing whether the disease was inside a woman's body, a result of her life of prostitution; these women could contract incurable cases of the French disease.[141] Although Venice's response to the French disease from the sixteenth century to the eighteenth century had shifted from beauty to poverty, the focus remained on women's bodies as sources of disease and women's behavior as an object of moral reform. Judging from the large marketplace for French disease cures throughout Europe, this approach had limited impact.[142]

The Incurables hospital and female asylums were part of a wider European trend during the late sixteenth century in which charitable institutions played a role not only in providing services to the poor and indigent classes, but also in developing methods of controlling and disciplining the poor through efforts to reform and correct their behavior. In contrast to informal social control, such as neighborhood gossip, "social disciplining" refers to the formal processes (enacted in laws and the creation of institutions) in which both church and state authorities tried to change their subjects' behavior to establish order and strengthen societies, often at the expense of newly marginalized sub-populations who were increasingly subject to a variety of punishments. The "social disciplining" model has become so popular for explaining the growth of sixteenth-century poor laws and charitable institutions that scholars have recently cautioned about its overuse. Early modern reformers' goal was often to rehabilitate rather than merely punish certain disaffected groups, and the early modern state often lacked the power and resources to control their populations.[143] Furthermore, certain groups, even relatively stigmatized groups such as sodomites, sometimes successfully resisted efforts to control them.[144] The impact of Michel Foucault's work in particular during the 1980s and 1990s led to what many scholars regard as an exaggerated emphasis on the power of the early modern state and its attempt to confine and control certain sub-populations.[145]

Nonetheless, because of widespread attempts by local governments and by both Protestant and Catholic institutions to reform behavior through charitable works, the idea of "social disciplining" during this period is still a useful concept, if not overstated in terms of the coherence, unity, and power of early modern states.[146] From the perspective of the women who found the female asylums too stifling, "social disciplining" was precisely what they seem to have encountered and found objectionable within these institutions. The female asylums changed over time precisely because they did not have the financial resources and power to impose order on their "target audience" of fallen women or beautiful, impoverished young girls. Charitable institutions in Venice and throughout the Italian peninsula were enmeshed in wider patron–client relationships that forced these institutions to adapt to patrons' requests and needs, including practical motivations such as securing lodging for a relative or friend, or overseeing the enforcement of patrons' last wills and testaments.[147] Men entered into the hospital for French disease treatment, for a limited period, primarily to receive the highly valued guaiacum treatment.

Like medical care outside of institutions, institutional health care in early modern Venice represents a mixed legacy. On the one hand, they provided services that French disease patients and their families demanded: affordable guaiacum treatments, shelter, and a means of survival. On the other hand, these institutions reinforced gender prejudices by holding women accountable for the French disease and requiring them to be lifetime penitents. Furthermore, the early female asylums demanded a complete change of life, including physical removal from families and friends, with only the possibility of limited, supervised visits. Little wonder that these early female asylums failed to fulfill their mandate. More surprising is that Venetian authorities in the eighteenth century continued to focus on female penitence as one strategy for controlling the French disease, despite more than a century of failure with that approach.

Conclusion

On November 18, 1616, Giovanni Battista Indorado presented a petition to the Venetian government requesting the authority to raise his nephew and two nieces and safeguard their remaining assets for their future, because his sister and her husband were too ill with the French disease to be able to raise the children themselves. With the couple confined to their beds due to the extremity of their illness, the family had fallen into poverty, having sold all of their furniture and razed their fields, selling even the stones from the field and the wooden doors and balcony of their house. The three children, Pietro, Anzola, and Giulia, possessed only one shirt each and no shoes, thereby forced to go about half-naked and barefooted. Their uncle claimed that neither the medical arts nor medications had been able to restore his sister Isabella to health, whose illness he claimed she had acquired from her husband.[1] Although it is impossible to determine how Isabella acquired her illness, what is important is the evidence of the real suffering that the French disease could and did inflict on families and communities in early modern Venice and throughout Europe.[2] For the majority of Venetians who were not wealthy, the French disease brought a double-blow: incapacitating illness and accompanying financial hardship or even poverty.

This book has drawn attention to the importance of studying the French disease as an endemic disease in early modern Venice. Although most scholarly attention has focused on the initial epidemic, the shift to endemic disease has been comparatively neglected and is important for a variety of reasons. As an endemic rather than epidemic disease, the French disease threatened more people and reached more broadly into the population. First associated with wartime's mobile soldiers and camp followers, the French disease accompanied them home and stayed, spreading to lovers, spouses, and also children. Venice's relatively mobile residents facilitated the transmission of disease. Countryside and city were linked through seasonal migration, while different neighborhoods were linked through common social ties. Venice's multiple bridges linked the city's diverse neighborhoods, with common meeting points at the Rialto market and nearby piazzas. Venice's elite marriage practices contributed to the development of a sexual culture in which sexual relationships between elites and commoners were fairly common and tolerated, as long as these relationships did not end in marriage. A variety of regular activities—the employment of domestic servants, renting of rooms to migrants, attendance at church or market, and the cultivation of patron–client ties in business—provided multiple avenues for people of different ethnicities (Greek, Istrian, Tuscan, and so forth) and social classes to meet and, in some cases, become lovers or sexual partners.

In its epidemic phase, the French disease was initially spread primarily by soldiers, prostitutes, and their immediate partners. But the situation changed dramatically when the disease became endemic. Soldiers and prostitutes did not have a monopoly on the French disease. As a common disease, infiltrating every *sestieri*, social class and status group, including the clergy, Venetians could potentially contract the French disease from just about anyone: their spouses, their long-term lovers, or their fellow tenant with whom they shared an apartment and other intimacies, among others. Widespread sexual violence brought the French disease to its victims, while sexual coercion—the employer seeking sexual favors from a domestic servant, for example—also played a role in transmitting disease. A young woman hoping to avoid the French disease could not simply decide not to work as a prostitute and remain safe: she might contract the disease from her husband, her long-time lover whom she hoped to marry, or from a rapist.

Who is primarily responsible for the spread of disease and who is primarily at risk to become newly infected are different for epidemic and endemic disease. This fundamental difference has important implications for the prevention and control of sexually transmitted diseases, including HIV/AIDS. In new epidemics that are concentrated among sub-populations, such as sex workers or injecting drug users, prevention efforts are most effective when they target these particular groups. When the disease has spread to become a "generalized epidemic" or endemic disease, the tactics and targets must change as well.[3]

Furthermore, even in epidemics, prostitutes and their partners are not necessarily the major engines driving the epidemic. In early modern Venice, the word *meretrice* encompassed women in many different circumstances, basically referring to any woman who engaged in sexual relations outside of marriage. Because Venice was a regional hub of migration, the city attracted many unmarried men and women. Unmarried women faced challenging prospects for securing long-term security: skilled jobs were out of their reach because of guilds' restrictions on training, while legitimate marriage required a dowry which many working-class women lacked. In such an unstable environment, informal sexual relationships flourished. The early modern Venetian situation bears some similarities to that of the Central African Republic and the city of Kinshasa in the Democratic Republic of Congo (DRC), where the HIV/AIDS epidemics were not primarily the product of relations between prostitutes and their clients. In Kinshasa, widespread female unemployment combined with the common practice of taking concubines and relative "sexual freedom" were the major factors behind the HIV/AIDS epidemic, which, despite its seriousness, never reached the level that it attained in Kigali, Rwanda, where keeping a concubine was a less common practice. Kigali's epidemic, by contrast, emerged primarily as the result of married men's sexual relations with prostitutes and subsequent infection of their wives with HIV. These differences in sexual culture influenced the patterns of infection in Kinshasa and Kigali: in Kigali, women aged 25–35 are most likely to be infected, whereas in Kinshasa young women and older men are infected.[4] In early modern Venice, like Kinshasa, sexuality was hardly restricted to the marital bed and the brothel. The lack of reliable prevalence data prevents making more of a comparison between Venice and modern African cities, but the overall comparison with Kinshasa and its sexual openness is nonetheless suggestive.

The prostitute was nonetheless a potent symbol of the French disease in early modern Venice. In a city that was often represented as a beautiful woman in the figure of either the Virgin Mary or the sensual Venus, goddess of love, the image of a disease-ridden prostitute carried enormous symbolic weight. Beauty represented God's grace on the serene city-state of Venice, but also its potential attraction and vulnerability to foreign invaders. One mid-sixteenth-century popular medical treatise recounted the story of how a beautiful woman captured the attentions of the invading French army in the late fifteenth century; intercourse with so many men caused the mixing of all their seed within her body and subsequent creation and spread of the French disease. This story incorporated Renaissance literary tropes about the dangers of female beauty and reinforced the perception that uncontrolled female sexuality represented a threat to Venice's political and military security.

The Italian Wars had ushered in a period of constant interference from major European powers in Italian politics, while the growing power of the Turks presented danger from the east in particular to the Venetian republic. In the wake of past military defeats during the Italian Wars and ongoing threats from the Turks, Venetians expressed anxieties about the military strength and discipline of their fighting men. The French disease represented masculine weakness as well as the dangers of the female sex. Early modern Italian writers lamented the inability of Italian soldiers to resist the distractions of the fair sex. Italian masculinity was not what it had once been in the days of the Roman Republic, when disciplined soldiers could resist the temptations of a beautiful woman. Titian's 1560 painting of *Mars, Venus, and Amor* illustrates a certain ambivalence toward the pleasures of Venus, as the love-struck Mars removes his armor in order to make love to Venus. Well-known as a city of love and pleasure, famed for its beautiful courtesans, Venice was also vulnerable to attack during the sixteenth century. The French disease served as a potent warning of the dangers of indiscipline by men and women alike to the continued stability of the Republic.

The French disease therefore bore considerable symbolic weight as a sign of military decline and vulnerability. Despite differences in medical and popular opinion about where the disease ultimately originated, whether it was entirely new or an older disease returned, or whether the result of cannibalism, a conjunction of the planets, or sexual intercourse between a prostitute and soldiers which sparked an epidemic, all agreed that the disease at least coincided with the French invasion of Italy and the subsequent humiliations of the Italian Wars (1494–1530). A focus on the French invasion did not abate with time, as the Italian peninsula never regained its autonomy and strength. On the contrary, by the mid-sixteenth century the French invasion came to be seen as the turning point in the political and military history of the Italian city-states, as Florence and Milan fell to Habsburg power. The French disease was a visible sign of political and military vulnerability, a continuing weakness in the face of ever-greater Turkish strength. The stigma associated with the French disease was reproduced during the period because it was associated with the sexuality or immoral behavior of individuals, but also because of the potential impact of that behavior on the political strength of the society as a whole. The French disease literally embodied Italian vulnerability. Outside of Italy, the French disease or the "pox" carried an equally rich set of meanings. From Shakespeare's *Timon of Athens* to Rabelais's *Pantagruel*, the pox appeared frequently in literature and plays far more often than any disease except the plague itself.[5]

The transition from epidemic to endemic disease brought about a shift in how patients experienced illness and how the public perceived the disease. As an epidemic disease, the French disease signified collective moral failure, God's punishment for sin. Preachers like Girolamo Savonarola criticized the vanity and worldliness of the Florentines. Patients faced the disease with little confidence in a cure. As an endemic, curable disease, however, the disease became something that had to be managed but did not inspire as much fear. Blame shifted to the individual patient, especially in cases of apparently incurable illness.

Although the French disease was never considered easy to treat and might initially persist despite treatment, physicians and much of the public regarded the disease as ultimately curable if properly managed through diet, exercise, medicines, and perhaps spiritual care. The kind of treatment that patients sought depended upon a host of factors, especially their resources, but also their gender. The French disease bore greater stigma for female than male patients, but even men did not always escape blame and shame. Men and women could consult advice books and purchase medications directly from pharmacies without revealing their condition to a medical practitioner; a few books specifically targeted female patients and discreetly offered advice for those suffering from the French disease and other potentially embarrassing ailments. Popular healers provided medical care to French patients and allowed for the possibility that bewitchment, rather than immoral behavior, was the cause of disease. Many patients seem to have found that approach attractive, based on the numbers of popular healers selling cures and offering treatment. Unlike in England, however, university-trained physicians were comfortable treating French-disease patients, so that treatment of this disease was not primarily handled by popular healers.

Resolutely incurable cases of the disease led university-trained physicians to suspect that the patients were somehow to blame, either because they had been unusually sinful and not truly penitent, or had simply failed to follow doctor's orders. Patient's families, however, interpreted treatment failure differently: they suspected witchcraft in cases of incurable disease. Since the Holy Office formally investigated cases of suspected witchcraft and relied on physicians' expert testimony, however, not a single accusation of practicing witchcraft to infect someone with the French disease stood up in court. No one in early modern Venice received a guilty verdict for maliciously causing a French disease case via witchcraft. Although that is certainly a happy outcome to point out, the reality was a bit more complex. Suspected witches were not blamed for treatment failures, but patients were. Physicians' testimony inevitably hinged on the patients' moral failings as the reason for their inability to respond to treatment. The medical treatments themselves, however, including the guaiacum, various unguents, diet, and exercise regimens, were not questioned.

As a common disease, the French disease had therefore become somewhat routine in early modern Venice and incapable of provoking the wider scientific and philosophical debates it had engendered as an epidemic disease. Physicians, empirics, and popular healers were quite content to continue offering the same medicines and advice and peddling the same cures during the late sixteenth and seventeenth centuries, with minor variations on the same ingredients. What is surprising is that no one realized something was amiss: large numbers of people were regularly becoming infected and dying without receiving effective treatment, but that went unnoticed. The complex system of medical treatments, along with the French disease's apparently intermittent nature (a trait it shares with modern venereal syphilis, which of course it might very well be), conspired to render the large dimensions of this tragedy invisible. The French disease or the pox was certainly still an important literary and moral theme, but it was no longer a medically interesting question.

Hospitals and institutional care were a crucial part of Venice's response to the French disease. Because of the large numbers of people too sick to work and gradually becoming impoverished from illness, Venice and other major Italian cities were forced to come up with solutions to the problem of the chronically ill. Victims of the bubonic plague did not linger, of course, and require long-term care. The French disease thereby strained existing hospitals and institutions, primarily oriented to epidemic disease or acute illness. Inspired and even led by key Counter-Reformation orders, Italian cities gave permission to found "Incurables" hospitals primarily for those suffering from the French disease, or other chronic, incurable illnesses. Even when the French disease came to be regarded as curable, however, the institutional separation between chronic, endemic diseases and acute, epidemic diseases remained, because treatment for the French disease required weeks or even months of care.

Hospitals provided care to greater numbers of male than female patients, despite apparently equal rates of infection. Gender distinctions were central to the institutional care provided in Venice. Two female asylums arose within the Incurables hospitals and specifically targeted French disease patients or young girls considered to be at risk of defilement and hence at risk of becoming French disease patients. These female asylums reinforced the perception that women were the ultimate cause of disease. Furthermore, while male patients could be easily reintegrated into society after receiving medical and spiritual care at the hospital, female patients were not perceived as candidates fit for immediate reintegration into society. At the Convertite, women were encouraged to take life-long vows of penitence as nuns in the Augustinian order.

In practice and over time, however, the female asylums (the Convertite and the Zitelle) no longer served their founding purpose as part of a plan to prevent sexual defilement or provide a refuge and place of penitence for women sexually active outside of marriage and thereby reduce the impact of the French disease on society. Because there was such a strong demand for institutions that provided security, literacy, and spiritual life to women and girls of the working and artisan classes, the institutions' governors bent the rules and admitted people who did not strictly conform to the rules for admission. In addition, women who did fulfill the conditions for entry did not necessarily want to spend the remainder of their lives in perpetual penitence. During the seventeenth century, these female asylums ceased to play a role as part of Venice's response to the French disease and instead became repositories for women who could not easily integrate into Venetian society for a variety of reasons: they might have been rape victims, estranged wives, or pious working-class virgins who could not afford to enter a traditional convent. In the eighteenth century, however, Venetian political and church officials renewed their interest in female asylums as part of an integrated response to the French disease. A new female asylum, the Penitenti, was created, with a new focus. Rather than targeting beautiful women and girls as being particularly vulnerable to the French disease, the Penitenti targeted impoverished women. As part of the Enlightenment emphasis on alleviating poverty and other social ills, Venetian social reformers emphasized poverty, not beauty, as at risk of contracting the French disease. Although reformers shifted their emphasis from beauty to poverty, they nonetheless continued to target females for institutional care and encourage their penitence. The Penitenti's ultimate goal, however, was not the permanent removal of these women from society, but their ultimate reintegration as domestic servants and workers in Venice's economy.

This study has highlighted the many ways in which the experience of endemic disease differed from epidemic disease at the social, cultural, medical, and institutional levels. Gender has been a central theme because of the important role it played in integrating the French disease into Venetian culture and institutions. The danger of female bodies was already an important trope in early modern Italian culture. Linking the French disease to female bodies became a way of making the French disease more familiar and less threatening to Venetians, in the same way that similarity to leprosy was highlighted in the epidemic phase to make the new disease seem less strange and disruptive. The establish-ment of female asylums thereby reassured early modern Venetians that female sexuality was now under control and hence less of a threat to Venice's stability. Until the end of the eighteenth century, Venetians continued to focus on the control of female sexuality as a key element to the control of the French disease.

Afterword

On Wednesday, September 16, 2009, the daily newspaper *The Ghanaian Times* reported an all too-common occurrence. According to the newspaper, a 57-year-old man who has been living with HIV for 17 years was told by his pastor that he had been cured of HIV "and then assured him it was not necessary to visit a clinic." Another woman reported that her pastor gave her bottles of anointed oil to drink until she vomited, then told her that she had vomited the virus. Confident that she was no longer sick, she unknowingly passed the virus to her unborn son who subsequently died; a trip to a local public clinic or hospital would have enabled her to undergo a relatively simple and effective treatment to prevent transmission of the virus to her unborn child.

> 'The problem we have in this country is that we are God-fearing people,' [she] said. 'Any problem we have we take it to God, so whatever the pastor says, we do. Some people are convinced that if [you] pray or if [you] do this without the antiretroviral drugs, you will be cured. But if God will cure me, it will surely come from above and not the pastor.'[1]

This newspaper account is only one of many reports in Ghana and throughout sub-Saharan Africa of widespread and persistent beliefs that HIV/AIDS is a spiritual disease, caused by witches or by God's punishment for sin, and therefore cured through spiritual means.[2] Trained as scientists, public health officials are often reluctant to engage directly with the religious dimension of people's perceptions of HIV/AIDS. Their reluctance is understandable, given that serious misunderstanding could result if the public thought that their religious beliefs were being criticized or attacked by health officials. But ignoring the religious dimensions of people's perceptions of HIV/AIDS allows some misperceptions to exist and limits the public's willingness to access life-saving care and treatment. This is where history becomes useful. The historical example of Venice, coping with a sexually transmitted disease during a period of intense religious expression and widespread belief in witchcraft, bears some similarity to many countries or regions within Africa. Much of Africa is currently undergoing a religious revival, especially of charismatic and evangelical Christianity, Catholic as well as Protestant. It would be useful if more African leaders, especially those in areas with large Christian populations, became familiar with the long history of Christian responses to sexually transmitted diseases as natural illnesses, treatable by doctors through medications. Venice's past experience with the French disease not only provides important insights for the present global struggle to control HIV/AIDS, but also for other sexually transmitted diseases and commonly stigmatized endemic illnesses. In this afterword, I will highlight three areas in which insights for the present can be drawn: (1) blame and witchcraft accusations; (2) the relative neglect of sexually transmitted diseases due to stigma and the availability of effective therapeutics; and (3) prevention as a tool to keep epidemic diseases from becoming endemic.

Christianity and belief in witchcraft currently coexist in much of Africa. As anthropologists have recently shown, witchcraft beliefs in Africa are not necessarily relics of "traditional" religion; in fact, belief in witchcraft has shown tremendous vitality in periods of modernization, and the beliefs and practices have changed over time.[3] In sub-Saharan Africa, patients and communities often accuse individuals of having caused AIDS through the practice of witchcraft, a belief system that protects the patient from the social stigma associated with sexual acquisition of disease.[4] There is no reason to believe that these witchcraft accusations are cynical attempts to manage stigma rather than expressions of belief in both the physical and spiritual causes of illness, much as was the case in early modern Venice.

Venetian physicians protected those accused of witchcraft from potential harm by insisting that the disease was of natural rather than supernatural origins. As expert witnesses for the Holy Office, Venetian physicians were operating within a framework that accepted the idea of supernatural causation of disease. They did not attack the fundamental beliefs of ordinary people; instead, they shared these beliefs and instead argued that these specific cases did not involve witchcraft. In modern South Africa, however, the courts that investigate the witchcraft accusations operate with the assumption that witchcraft does not exist and therefore these courts often lack popular legitimacy. The public often believes that the courts allow guilty witches to get off scot-free.[5] The solution is, of course, not to bring back the Holy Office of the Inquisition. But it is worth exploring how spiritual and biomedical approaches to disease prevention and control could be combined in order to address public perceptions of spiritual causes of illness. Christian pastors and priests need to understand that, historically, Christian leaders acknowledged the role of medicine in the treatment of sexually transmitted diseases. Religion and medicine were complementary, not competing, responses to illness. Careful, planned training of an incorporation of traditional healers and religious leaders from all major religions into HIV/AIDS prevention and care programs may provide one avenue for a simultaneous struggle against witchcraft accusations and AIDS-related stigma.[6]

Stigma is a difficult and complex issue. As Susan Sontag famously noted, illness serves as a powerful metaphor during any age. The metaphoric associations of a given illness make the experience of that illness more difficult, she argued

> My point is that illness is *not* a metaphor, and that the most truthful way of regarding illness—and the healthiest way of being ill—is one most purified of, most resistant to, metaphoric thinking.[7]

Sontag documented the ways in which the metaphors of illness made the experience of living with cancer and other diseases much more difficult: these metaphors contributed to the stigmatization of disease. She also recommended that societies try to purge themselves of this tendency to use disease as a metaphor.

Given the ubiquity with which illness, not only sexually transmitted diseases but also leprosy, mental illness, and epilepsy, becomes stigmatized and embedded in larger discourses about gender, social relations, power, morality, and even political and military strength, it might be useful to pause for a moment and ask whether Sontag's strategy of combating metaphors is the most useful approach to reduce disease-related stigma. Most public health interventions that have attempted to reduce, for example, HIV/AIDS stigma have taken Sontag's approach in trying to replace cultural associations of disease with correct medical knowledge about how HIV is transmitted.[8] Stigma is one of the major problems for patients with HIV/AIDS, which impacts their ability to access care and treatment. Stigma also impedes prevention, when people are unwilling to discuss a disease because of perceptions of stigma.[9] But the approach of combating stigma with correct knowledge operates on the assumption that stigma is simply incorrect knowledge, an idea challenged by recent work on stigma. Correct knowledge about how HIV is transmitted does help reduce stigma by reducing fear of transmission through casual contact, but it is not sufficient on its own. Stigma is embedded in broader patterns of power and domination: to understand how stigma is created and reproduced, it is necessary to understand and confront social inequality in a given society.[10]

The way in which these new insights about stigma can be translated into practical programs to combat stigma in communities is suggested by the work of an anthropologist, Sarah Castle, on HIV/AIDS stigma in Mali. She quoted two different informants' explanation of the origin and transmission of AIDS via young Malians who migrate to Côte d'Ivoire contract HIV/AIDS:

> This is what I have heard. I myself was in Côte d'Ivoire and even saw a child who was with a white person and who slept with a dog. They say that she became infected by the dog. If these girls come and sleep with our young men, that's how they get AIDS. That is the information I have.
>
> (Village A, father of out-of-school girl, 54 years old (FGD))

> AIDS? Aagh! [laughs] it is the illness of dogs. Because white people get their dogs ready and then suggest to girls who are looking for money—large sums of money—that they have sex with their dogs and so this is how they get AIDS. It is not an illness sent from God but from men and it is white people that have brought it to us. In this way they [the girls] come back, ever so charming, and they will seduce men easily—who in turn will be infected if they sleep together.
>
> (Village B, head of the hunters (gatekeeper), 90-year-old (IDI)).[11]

These descriptions of possible mechanisms of transmission elucidate a range of anxieties and perceived vulnerabilities: the economic vulnerability of young Malian females, forced to trade sex for money; the vulnerability of the Malian economy, whose workers migrate to neighboring Côte d'Ivoire to support themselves and families back home; the anxieties about corrupt and morally decadent whites, who still exercise political and economic influence in the post-colonial era. As with the case of Renaissance Venice, fear of biological contagion incorporates fears about other kinds of contagion: moral, cultural, political, and social. Castle underscored the importance of addressing the social context of infection, in addition to factual misperceptions about HIV transmission and acquisition, in developing interventions to reduce HIV/AIDS stigma. "In particular," she argues, "the community needs to openly confront fears about labour migration and the re-integration of returned migrants so that they can be accommodated sensitively within village life rather than reacted to with blame and mistrust."[12] Discussions about illness reveal underlying social fissures and tensions, which are projected onto a particular disease.

Disease origin and transmission stories thereby convey useful information about communities' perceptions of their own vulnerabilities, especially those they perceive as threats to the public health of their communities. Historical and ethnographic analyses play an important role in efforts to reduce stigma by learning more about which groups are perceived as vulnerable and why, and which groups require more support. Public health interventions can dramatically reduce stigma, but these efforts are more effective when they engage communities meaningfully about their perceptions of disease and how they become entangled in perceptions of morality, shame, and blame.[13] It might be useful to think about how to develop public health conversations with local communities about political, social, and economic vulnerability to HIV/AIDS, and ways to reduce it.[14] Recent studies have shown that stigma can be reduced through programs that focus both on people's fear of infection through casual contact and through frank discussions about morals and values: it is important to dissociate the disease from behaviors considered to be immoral.[15] For example, a faithful person can contract HIV if his or her partner has or had other partners.

But Venice's example also provides an important warning about how physicians and others can increase stigma by blaming patients. Unfortunately, Venetian physicians placed the blame for treatment failure and death from disease squarely on the patient. Immoral patients died. In the present age of HIV/AIDS, blame for treatment failure is likely to take on a more subtle, but nonetheless insidious form: suggesting that patients whose health does not improve are at fault for not taking their medications regularly or properly. In fact, it is critically important for patients to take their regulations regularly and on time, or they run the risk of developing resistance to the medications. Worse yet, the HIV virus within their bodies, now resistant to the antiretroviral medications, can spread to others. Antiretroviral medications for resistant strains of HIV are not yet available in most of Africa: the costs are prohibitive. Patients who do not take their medications therefore threaten not only their own health, but also the health of others. It is certainly tempting to blame patients for their treatment failure, but wrong. Patients who carefully follow the instructions and take their medications on time may nonetheless develop resistance and fail to improve. But not all patients will respond to antiretroviral therapy, especially if, because of fear, stigma, or ignorance, the patient delayed seeking treatment until very late, as is often the case in sub-Saharan Africa. Furthermore, in developing countries, patients have access to only one or, if they are lucky, two types of treatment regimens; if they do not respond to treatment, which as many as between 12 percent and 15 percent of patients do not, they do not have recourse to another combination of drugs, as they might in a richer country.[16] In addition, approximately 25 percent of pregnant women who test positive and who have received a temporary course of Highly Active Antiretroviral Therapy (HAART) to prevent transmission of HIV to their babies develop drug-resistant strains of HIV within a year.[17] In this case, treatment failure would be the result of efforts to protect her unborn children from acquiring HIV, hardly an act of moral failure. The risk to women's health from short-term treatment has caused a few public health advocates to urge mandatory long-term treatment of these women for the sake of the their own health, in addition to that of their babies.[18] Blaming the patient for treatment failure is often wrong and usually counter-productive.

Secondly, this historical study of Venice is also intended as a reminder of the ongoing human suffering and problems that major diseases present, even when they come to be regarded as routine, as could happen with HIV/AIDS within this decade. The French disease continued to exact a heavy toll during the seventeenth century, but the public, including the authorities, largely ignored the disease once they regarded it as "contained" within the bodies of institutionalized women and controlled through a system of therapeutics. Ironically, the development of medical therapies that are accepted as effective—and, in their day, mercury and guaiacum were regarded as effective, in addition to a host of other remedies—can be deleterious to the overall control of disease. Public and official interest in and support for disease control can wane when new therapies become available.[19] It is a reminder that our commitment to the prevention, care, and treatment of major diseases such as HIV/AIDS and tuberculosis should not diminish, but intensify as effective therapies become available. No cure exists for HIV/AIDS, but antiretroviral therapy is effective in reducing mortality and improving health and quality of life for those infected.

The commonness and seriousness of a disease is no guarantee that public attention and resources will be devoted to it. Like in early modern Venice, sexually transmitted diseases are currently endemic in the US and also globally, but they are not a major focus of public concern, largely due to stigma. Only two journalists attended the release of a major report by the Institute of Medicine that highlighted the impact of sexually transmitted diseases on health in the US.[20] Bacterial sexually transmitted diseases continue to cause a major impact, while rates of viral STDs have increased worldwide. For example, the World Health Organization estimated that approximately 89 million new cases of genital chlamydial infection occurred in 2001; in the US in 2004, almost one million cases were reported, making it the most common reportable disease in the country.[21] Although the long-term health consequences of chlamydial infection are serious and include pelvic inflammatory disease, infertility, and Reiter's syndrome (arthritis) in adults and eye disease and pneumonia in infants born to infected mothers, efforts to reduce the disease have not received the necessary attention and resources, despite the fact that an effective curative treatment exists.[22]

Although HIV/AIDS has received the lion's share of attention in sub-Saharan Africa, it is by no means the only issue. Human papilloma virus (HPV) is another serious infection because of its role in the aetiology of cervical cancer. In fact, cervical cancer is the most common cancer among women in sub-Saharan Africa. Worldwide, over 80 percent of cervical cancer deaths occur in developing countries. Although a vaccine that is effective against the strains of HPV that are associated with cervical cancer is available, the vaccine's high cost currently limits access in developing countries. Furthermore, syphilis and gonorrhea remain ongoing problems worldwide, despite the availability of effective and affordable treatment. The reason why these diseases remain relatively neglected is, of course, their connection to sexuality, which brings us to our last point.

Venice's historical example provides insights into how to tackle one of the thorniest issues in the prevention of sexually transmitted diseases: how to confront the morally loaded topic of sexuality. Venetian officials made a tactical mistake that undermined their efforts to control disease. They blurred all distinctions between women who primarily earned their living through sale of sex versus unmarried women in a "love" relationship with a man who paid part of their expenses. These two groups had different perspectives. The latter often hoped for marriage or a stable relationship with their lover; they wanted to continue, not cut off, these relationships, and they did not regard themselves as prostitutes. Venice's Convertite required that these relationships end, thereby making the convent an unattractive option for many women. In addition, by emphasizing that the French disease was spread by prostitution, Venetian authorities contributed to the stigmatization of disease and thereby undermined control efforts.

The Venetian situation is eerily similar to that of sub-Saharan Africa, most of which suffers from the world's worst epidemic not because of prostitution alone, but because of the phenomenon known as "transactional sex." As Helen Epstein explains in her study of AIDS in East and southern Africa, transactional sex involves not just the exchange of goods and cash for sex, but also feelings; a relationship of some degree of intimacy develops. "Although transactional sex, like prostitution, involves the exchange of cash and other goods, the gifts themselves are often of less importance than the social connections and relationships they signify ... Like a kinship system, networks of transactional relationship provide a social security system for women and a source of power and self-esteem for men."[23]

Unfortunately, however, transactional sex can be even riskier than prostitution in terms of its risk of transmitting HIV. Because there is a certain degree of intimacy between partners, people are less likely to use condoms. In addition, people who practice transactional sex are also likely to carry on a few relationships *simultaneously* in which they do not use condoms, rather than successive relationships in which one relationship ends before another begins. That means that if one person becomes infected, the others are at risk: HIV is most infectious in the early stages before the person has even tested positive. They may not have as many total partners as someone who frequents brothels, but their risk of transmitting and acquiring HIV may in fact be higher because of the type of sexual network they have created. In sub-Saharan Africa, for example, people often have a lower lifetime number of partners than they do in industrialized, Western countries, but because they maintain these relationships simultaneously rather than successively they are at greater risk of transmitting sexually transmitted diseases.[24] Part of the reason that Uganda successfully reduced its prevalence of HIV is because of its "zero grazing" campaign, a locally developed slogan to reduce the number of sexual partners for both men and women.[25] No such attempt to reduce the number of sexual partners was made in Venice. While the authorities blamed prostitutes for the spread of disease, elite Venetian males continued to enjoy sexual relationships with several women, who themselves often practiced "transactional sex" as a survival strategy. The lesson is that prevention efforts need to be targeted toward the specific situation: epidemics primarily fueled by transactional sex require a different prevention and control strategy than those driven primarily by commercial sex.

On the positive side, however, Venetian authorities developed a few components of a useful model for responding to the needs of sex workers. They learned from their earlier mistakes with the Convertite that it was important to provide skills for former sex workers in order to reintegrate them into the economy. After the failures of the Convertite, the new Penitenti focused on training women and placing them in secure jobs so that they would not return to sex work. HIV/AIDS prevention and care programs targeted toward sex workers need to take account of the material and economic circumstances of their lives and offer resources that enable them to choose a different livelihood, rather than punish and isolate them. Although early modern Venetians continued to focus on women's bodies to control disease, they shifted toward less punitive practices during the eighteenth century and toward reintegration of "fallen women" into society. Unfortunately, however, this effort reached only a handful of women and was unlikely to have major impact on the spread of the French disease. Confident as they were in their ability to treat disease in patients defined as "normal," prevention was the most neglected aspect of Venice's response to the French disease.

Herein lies perhaps the most important lesson for the present: the importance of continuing to emphasize prevention. As antiretroviral medications have become increasingly available around the world, there is a danger of neglecting the prevention of HIV/AIDS. No longer necessarily a death sentence (though millions still die every year), AIDS has become less scary. People who were once scared are taking risks again, as the increase in syphilis cases among gay men in San Francisco and other urban centers in the first decade of 2000 indicates.[26] History teaches us that sexual transmission remains an excellent means for a pathogen to spread through a population, and that new, as yet undiscovered organisms, are likely to travel along that pathway. We are far from actually having controlled HIV/AIDS, and we are not immune to the potential development of a new sexually transmitted disease. History reminds us that we need not face future threats unprepared: we have learned a lot about how sexually transmitted diseases spread through populations. By emphasizing prevention, especially appropriate prevention strategies for a given population, transformation of epidemics of sexually transmitted diseases into endemic diseases can be precluded. We have the tools to contain new epidemics of sexually transmitted diseases, as long as we have the courage and commitment to use these tools quickly and thoroughly.

Notes

Introduction

Part of this introduction has been revised and adapted from McGough and Erbelding, 2006, pp. 183–95.

1. For a general introduction to the Italian Wars, see Hay and Law, 1989, pp. 158–68; for a general discussion of the sack of Rome and its impact, see Cochrane, 1988, pp. 7–18.
2. For a collection of early primary sources on the French disease from throughout Italy, see Alfonso Corradi, "Nuovi Documenti per la storia delle malattie veneree in Italia della fine del '400 alla metà del '500," *Rendiconti* 4: 14–15 Milan, 1871: 1–32. See also Arrizabalaga, Henderson, and French, 1997.
3. Benedetti, 1549, p. 29. On ideas about pollution and contamination, see Douglas, 2002.
4. *I Diarii di Marin Sanuto*, 1878–1903, p. 47; pp. 288–9. *"Item, che Paulo Vitelli ha mal franzoso assai …. Et come dominio Alvosio Valaresso havia mal franzoso; voria danari per dar a la compagnia, dicendo non havia auto paga et si vedea disperato."*
5. Cited by Corradi, pp. 22–3.
6. Arrizabalaga, Henderson, and French, 1997, p. 50.
7. McNeill, 1998 revised edition, original 1977, pp. 232, 220–1; on syphilis, see also McNeill, 1972, 122–60.
8. A useful starting place for the vast literature on the social construction of illness is Lachmund and Stollberg, 1992; Rosenberg and Golden, 1992; Roy Porter's work provides wonderful examples of the application of this theoretical orientation in specific times and places, for example, Porter and Rousseau, 1998. Works of medical anthropology that have been particularly useful in helping me understand cultural responses to sexually transmitted disease are Farmer, 1992 and Hyde, 2007.
9. Arrizabalaga, Henderson, and French, 1997.
10. A useful introduction to early modern perceptions of illness and disease is Lindemann, 2006, pp. 8–12.
11. Arrizabalaga, Henderson, and French, 1997, pp. 259–67.
12. Foa, 1990, pp. 26–45.
13. Foa, 1990; Cady, 2005, pp. 159–86.
14. On Venetians' perception of the disruptive power of passion, see Ruggiero, 1993, pp. 88–129.
15. Hewlett, 2005, pp. 239–60; for the preoccupation with sodomy in Tuscany, see Rocke, 1996.
16. Hentschell, 2005, pp. 133–57; Harris, 1998; Harris, 2004.
17. The ways in which sexually transmitted diseases were social constructed in Europe changed over time. For example, syphilis became a symbol of sexual and alcoholic excess, a symptom of the stresses of modern urban living in late

nineteenth and early twentieth century Britain. Syphilis was considered to be one of the diseases of "civilization." See G. Davis, 2008, pp. 204–5.

18. Siena, 2004, p. 150.
19. Siena, 2004, pp.13, 115.
20. On the Zitelle, see Chojnacka, 1998, pp. 68–91, and Lionello, 1994; on all of the female communities, see Chojnacka, 2001, pp. 121–37 and Pullan, 1971; on the *Soccorso*, see Rosenthal, 1992, pp. 131–2; on the Convertite, see McGough, 1997. On these institutions in other Italian cities, see Cohen, 1992; Ferrante, 1990; Ciammitti, 1979, pp. 760–4; on Rome, see Groppi, 1994, and Camerano, 1993, pp. 227–60.
21. On the institutional link between hospitals for French disease patients and female asylums, see Arrizabalaga, French, and Henderson, 1997, p. 168; O'Malley, 1993, pp. 32–3; Pullan, 1971, pp. 377–8; Nordio, 1993/4, p. 128; Nordio, 1994.
22. The literature on cultural responses to epidemic disease is vast. A useful starting place is Ranger and Slack, 1996; an excellent example of a cultural study of chronic disease is Porter and Rousseau, 1998.
23. An exception is Hyde's *Eating Spring Rice*, in which she discusses "how HIV/ AIDS becomes embedded in political and economic relations, embodied practices, and cultural imaginations," p. 2.
24. See notes 8, 11, 12, 14 and 15.
25. For an interesting study of how an "invisible" disease, sickle cell anemia, became "visible" due to political, economic, and medical changes, see Wailoo, 2001.
26. One important exception is Schleiner, 1994, pp. 499–517; Kevin Siena is also attentive to gender issues in his *Venereal Disease, Hospitals, and the Urban Poor*. Gender analysis has been central to studies of modern venereal disease, however; a useful starting point is Spongberg, 1997.
27. Crawford, 2006, pp. 412–33.
28. On methodology, see especially Davis, 1987; Muir, 1991, pp. vii–xxviii. For an excellent example of how criminal records can be used to study sexuality, see Ruggiero, 1985.
29. For an excellent discussion of how "structural factors" such as opportunities to earn income can influence behavior and disease risk, see the discussion on "risk regulators" in Glass and McAtee, 2006.
30. The history of venereal diseases has often been studied in relation to the control of prostitution. Several works include Bernstein, 1995; Walkowitz, 1980; Corbin, 1990; Gibson, 1986.
31. Brandt, 1987, p. 167.
32. For an excellent discussion of the impact of the laboratory on conceptions of disease, see Cunningham, 2002, pp. 209–44.
33. Wilson, 2002, pp. 271–319.
34. On the problem of retrospective diagnosis with regard to the French disease, see Arrizabalaga, Henderson, and French, 1997, pp. 1–3; 17–18.
35. On Savonarola, see Weinstein, 1970; Arrizabalaga, Henderson, and French, 1997, p. 44.
36. Arrizabalaga, Henderson, and French, 1997, pp. 52–3.
37. Foreigners filled the ranks of infantry constables, while "large numbers of Albanian stradiots and even Turks were being used as light cavalry." Mallett, 1974, p. 232.
38. Mallett, 1984, pp. 56, 132–5.

39. On geographical origins, see McGough and Erbelding, 2006; Foa, 1990; Crosby, 1972, pp. 122–64. Other useful general studies of early modern syphilis include Buehrer, 1990, pp. 197–214 and Quétel, 1990.

40. Harper et al., 2008. For critical commentary from other scientists, see Mulligan et al., 2008.

41. Arrizabalaga, Henderson, and French, 1997.

42. Cipolla, C. (1970) "I Libri dei Morti," *Le Fonti della Demografia Storica in Italia* (Rome: CISP) Vol. I, Pt. II, 851–66; Cipolla, 1976, pp. 11–18; on bills of mortality in Italy, see p. 31.

43. It is not possible to determine the date of the first death attributed to the French disease, since the records between 1495 and 1503 are missing. Carmichael, 1991, pp. 187–200.

44. Baker and Armelagos, 1988, pp. 703–37. It is important to point out once again, however, that early modern perceptions of disease differed dramatically from modern perceptions. "Before the laboratory it was accepted that patients suffered from 'mixed' diseases, and that the 'morbid matter' freely moved within the body, which implied that any disease could change its seat, and even be transformed into another one" (Arrizabalaga, 1999, pp. 241–60, on p. 249). It was therefore possible for a case of leprosy to transform into a case of the French disease. For a specific case of early modern clinical diagnosis of the transformation of the French disease into leprosy, see Stein, 2006, pp. 617–48, on 617–8.

45. Laughran, 1998, p. 68.

46. Muir and Ruggiero, 1994, pp. vii–xviii; Davis, 1987; Rosaldo, 1986, pp. 77–97.

47. During the early sixteenth century, people more often used organic metaphors of the "body politic" to explain and understand the nature of politics. A body politic, as an organic entity, could suffer from ill health in a number of ways: internal corruption, threat of war from abroad, disruptive epidemics of plague or an outbreak of famine. For a particularly lucid explanation of the body politic metaphor in the Venetian context, see Laughran, October 17, 2002. Sperling, 1999, pp. 72–114.

48. Qualtiere and Slights 2003, pp. 1–23.

49. Parker and Aggleton, 2003, pp. 15–24. Link and Phelan, 2001, pp. 363–85.

50. Cohen, 1992.

1 A Network of Lovers: Sexuality and Disease Patterns in Early Modern Venice

1. *Candide*, 1990, pp. 9–10.

2. Morris, Goodreau, and Moody, 2008, p. 109–26.

3. The French disease was one of the most common ailments treated by Girolamo Cardano during the 1530s; most of his patients were from Milan, but he had also practiced in Venice, Sacco, Pavia, Bologna, and Rome. See Siraisi, 1997, p. 34. Similarly, David Gentilcore explains how the French disease was common enough throughout Italy to provide a steady stream of patients to both surgeons and physicians. See Gentilcore 2005, pp. 57–80.

4. On doctors who worked for the Sanità, see Carmichael, 1998; Cipolla, 1976, pp. 851–66. For the relationship between doctor and the state in Venice, see Ruggiero, 1978, pp. 156–84. On the strengths and limitations of mortality data as a source for Italian history, see Cipolla, 1970.

5. Arrizabalaga, 1999, pp. 241–60.
6. McGough, 2005, pp. 211–37; Siena, 2004, pp. 30–61.
7. City-wide population surveys in Venice typically do not include as many births and deaths as parish records, but not all parish records have survived. For the limitations on the study of Venetian demography, see Favero et al., 1991, pp. 23–110.
8. The state archives of Venice, Italy (Archivio di Stato di Venezia, henceforth ASV), Prov. alla Sanitá, Necrologi, Busta numbers 814–23, 834–41, 850–4, 867–70.
9. For example, in 1586, there were 16 deaths attributed to the French disease (bustas 817–18); in 1610, there were 14 deaths (bustas 840–1), while in 1638 there were only nine (bustas 868–9). ASV, Prov. alla Sanitá, Necrologi.
10. Arrizabalga et al., 1997, pp. 193, 187.
11. ASV, Ospitali et Luoghi Pii, Diversi, Busta 1031, Notatorio, f. 78r, f. 116r.
12. Siena, 2004, pp. 111–16.
13. Chojnacka, 2000, pp. 6–25.
14. ASV, Proved. alla Sanità, Busta numbers 814–23, 834–41, 850–4, 867–70.
15. ASV, Proved. alla Sanità, Busta 819, November 8, 1587; the patient was a 40-year-old wife of a carpenter; and Busta 815, October 5, 1583; the patient was a 48-year-old tailor.
16. For example, ASV, Proved. alla Sanità, Busta 815, December 5, 1583; this 40-year-old widow's illness was reported as having been only 15 days, but it is possible that the 15 days referred to fever, the other cause of death listed.
17. ASV, Prov. alla Sanità, Busta numbers 814–23, 834–41, 850–4, 867–70.
18. In medieval Bologna, Carol Lansing identified a gulf between social practice and elite definitions of female identity. While elite men could only define a woman as honest or a prostitute, people from working-class neighborhoods made many more distinctions, identifying several kinds of relationships outside of marriage, including a popularly accepted if not formal legal marriage. See Lansing, 2003, pp. 85–100.
19. On the ability of courtesans to attract male tourists, see Rosenthal, 1992, pp. 11–12; on sexual violence, see Ruggiero, 1985, pp. 89–108.
20. Davidson, 2002, pp. 65–81. On earlier repression of homosexual relations under the crime of sodomy and on the illicit culture of sexuality, see Ruggiero, 1985, pp. 109–45, 9–10. For the relationship between repression of sodomy and the Venetian state, see Chojnacki, 2000, pp. 32–7.
21. Davidson, "Sodomy in Early Modern Venice," p. 66.
22. The concern existed even before the Italian Wars, as Bernardo of Siena's sermons of the 1420s suggest when he advised wives to conceal their menstruation and engage in sex to keep their husbands from demanding anal intercourse. Rocke, 1998, pp. 150–70, on p. 156.
23. On Florence, see Rocke, 1996.
24. On the issue of homosexual identity, see the introduction to Chauncey, Duberman, and Vicinus, 1989, pp. 1–13.
25. Davidson, 2002, pp. 69–70.
26. Evidence of the relationships that ended with the woman's entry into the Convertite or Casa del Soccorso exists in the records of these institutions themselves, as well as the *Provveditori Sopra Monasteri, Processi Criminali*, and occasional trials in the *Sant'Uffizio*. See McGough, 1997.
27. Ferraro, 2001, pp. 106–17.

28. Cowan, 1999, pp. 276–93; Martini, 1986–7, pp. 305–26. Both examine the records of secret marriages from the patriarchal archives.
29. See notes 20 and 21. Ruggiero found extensive evidence of sexuality outside of marriage in Ruggiero, 1985, pp. 16–69.
30. On how to use criminal records as a source for social history, see the introduction to Muir and Ruggiero, 1994. I have borrowed from Natalie Davis about using these sources as evidence of acceptable cultural constructs in a given society and avoided, as Renato Rosaldo has argued, treating the Inquisitor or examining magistrate as an ethnographic fieldworker, providing notes in the form of a trial. See Davis, 1987; Renato Rosaldo, "From the Door of His Tent: The Fieldworker and the Inquisitor," in Clifford and Marcus, 1986, pp. 77–97.
31. *Parte presa nell'Eccellentissimo Conseglio di Pregadi*, February 21, 1542 m.v. (February 21, 1543).
32. Ferrante, 1986, pp. 51–3.
33. Dabhoiwala, 2001, pp. 85–8.
34. Klovdahl, 1985, pp. 1203 16, on p. 1210. After Klovdahl's article, there was a virtual explosion of interest in the application of social network theory to the AIDS epidemic. For early applications of the theory, see Anarfi and Awusabo-Asare, 1993, p. 1–15; *Sexually Transmitted Diseases* includes many articles on recent applications of social network theory, such as Boily et al., 2000, pp. 558–72. For a recent review of the literature on social networks and STD transmission, including HIV/AIDS, see Morris, Goodreau, and Moody, 2008, pp. 109–25.
35. Scott, 1991, p. 32.
36. Berkowitz, 1982, p. 2.
37. Klovdahl, 1985, p. 1203.
38. Klovdahl, 1985, p. 1203.
39. Wetherell, Plakans, and Wellman, 1994, p. 645. Charles Wetherell has been advocating the use of social network analysis since 1989. See Wetherell, 1989, pp. 645–51; Wellman and Wetherell, 1996, pp. 97–121; Wetherell, 1998, pp. 125–44. Aside from infectious diseases, Susan Cotts Watkins has shown the importance of social network analysis to explain changes in fertility patterns. See Watkins, 1995, pp. 295–311.
40. Barlow, 2001, p. 1458.
41. Gras et al., 1999, pp. 1953–62.
42. Campbell, 2003, pp. 28–31.
43. Lurie et al., 2003, pp. 149–56.
44. Lurie et al., 2003, pp. 2245–52.
45. The bibliography on patronage is vast, but an excellent starting place on the issue of the extent of patronage networks is Kent and Simons, 1987, especially chapters 2 and 5. For Venice, see Romano, 1987. His work concentrates on the fourteenth and fifteenth centuries. For the sixteenth and seventeenth centuries, see Davis, 1994, pp. 54–5, 135.
46. Romano, *Housecraft and Statecraft*, p. xv. Master–servant relationships were important throughout early modern Europe. For early modern France, for example, see Maza, 1983 and Fairchilds, 1984.
47. Chojnacka, 2000, pp. 6–25.
48. Zago, 1982.

49. Married noblewomen were often active patrons, especially of female kin, servants, and neighbors, in their immediate neighborhoods, so they were not completely socially isolated. See Romano, 1987. Nonetheless, out of fear of women's sexuality, noblewomen were closely monitored and not allowed free associations with other men, nor were they allowed freedom of movement throughout the city. See Romano, 1989, pp. 339–54, on pp. 347–8.
50. Chojnacka, pp. 81–6.
51. Molà, 2000, pp. 29–5.
52. The Sant'Uffizio records provide evidence of relationships which failed, since women often turned to love magic to try to win back their former lovers. See for example Sant'Uffizio, Busta 95, fasc. Bretti, Angela. Angela complained that her lover, Michiel de Morchi, a soldier posted to Padua, broke his promise to marry her and married a different women instead. It was possible to maintain more than one sexual relationship at a time. See also Ruggiero, pp. 30–1.
53. ASV, Sant'Uffizio, Busta 90, fasc. Fabri, Girolamo et al.
54. Overlapping sexual relationships are referred to as concurrent relationships in the literature on STDs and are associated with higher transmission rates through a population. See Morris, Goodreau, and Moody, 2008, pp. 117–20.
55. ASV, Sant'Uffizio, Busta 98, fasc. Fracnesca da Bari, denunciation of November 6, 1642 and testimony of Camilla, wife of Nicolai de Pipes, 40-year-old, December 16, 1642.
56. ASV, Sant'Uffizio, Busta 70, fasc. Felicita detta Greca, meretrice. Testimony of Ludovico, November 23, 1617. "lei non è maritata, lei ha ben un certo tal che la tiene chiamato Giulio dal Todesco." For similar cases, see Sant'Uffizio, Busta 73, fasc. Tommasina moglie di Nicolo barcaruol; Busta 81, fasc. Marioli Maria et al.
57. Cases sometimes came to court after man married a different woman and the abandoned woman allegedly practiced witchcraft against the new couple, the wife, or the man himself. See for example Sant'Uffizio, Busta 64, fasc. Azzalina, Livia; Sant'Uffizio, Busta 81, fasc. Marina Facchinetti and Lucia Bettinello; Sant'Uffizio, Busta 95, fasc. Bretti, Angela. The crime of defloration was also linked to failed expectations of marriage after the sexual act had occurred. Typically, the man promised to marry a woman and brought gifts to indicate his seriousness. He then failed to marry her, leaving her "deflowered" with diminished expectations of marriage. See Gambier, 1980; on defloration cases, Hacke, 2004, pp. 52–62; McGough, 1997, pp. 24–8; On women's ability to regain honor after losing virginity, see Ferrante, 1990, pp. 46–72.
58. Sant'Uffizio, Busta 81, fasc. Marina Facchinetti and Lucia Bettinello, testimony of February 26, 1626. "*Questo era mio moroso. Questo è quel che si è maritato questo Agosto. se bene mi haveva promesso di tuorme per moglie.*"
59. ASV, Sant'Uffizio, Busta 81, fasc. Marina Facchinetti, Lucia Bettinello, testimony of 26 Feb. 1626.
60. Concurrency has an exponential impact on the prevalence of STDs in a population. In Uganda in the early 1990s, for example, the HIV/AIDS prevalence doubled due to concurrent partnerships. Morris, Goodreau, and Moody, 2008, pp. 117–20.

61. Chojnacka, 2001, pp. 15–16.
62. Chojnacka, 2001, pp. 97–101.
63. The date was not recorded for 1642, although nearby San Martino was surveyed on April 14, 1642, so it was probably near that date. All of the censuses were taken in March and April of 1642.
64. All census data is from ASV, Prov. alla Sanità, Busta 570.
65. Chojnacka, 2001, p. 62.
66. Sperling, 1999, pp. 3, 19.
67. Davis, 1975; Chojnacki, 1990.
68. Sperling, 1999, p. 18.
69. Ruggiero, 1993; Eisenach, 2004.
70. Lane, 1973, pp. 254, 324.
71. Known as the "serrata" or closure of the Great Council. See Chojnacki, 1990, p. 117.
72. Pullan, 1971, pp. 228–9.
73. This idea is part of the so-called "myth of Venice." See Muir, 1981, pp. 13–61; Grubb, 1986, pp. 43–94.
74. Bottigheimer, 2002.
75. The literature on concubinage is vast, but an excellent starting place is Brundage, 1987.
76. Eisenach, 2004, pp. 146–7.
77. Ferraro, 2001, pp. 126–7.
78. See also Ruggiero, 2001, pp. 141–58.
79. The literature on the dowry system is vast. For Florence, see Klapisch-Zuber, 1985; Kirshner, 1978; Kuehn, 1991. Throughout Italy, see Cohn, 1996.
80. On dowry laws in Venice, see Ferro, 1845, pp. 641–3; also Bellavitis, 1998, pp. 91–100; Chojnacki, 1975, pp. 571–600.
81. Ambrosini, 2000, pp. 420–53, on pp. 434–5; on immigrant women in Venice, see Chojnacka, 2001, pp. 81–102.
82. The guilds formally restricted the kinds of opportunities open to women, thereby limiting women's ability to earn income on their own. Although women were allowed to be members if their fathers or husbands also were, women were not allowed to achieve the status of master and earned less than men. They were more likely to be found in the textile and clothing trades, along with trade in second hand goods. Even in these trades, however, their numbers were small. The mercers' guild, which sold haberdashery and dry goods of all types, listed 31 women among its 964 members, a little more than 3 percent of the total. Mackenney, 1987, pp. 23, 103. The situation in Bologna was similar; see Dumont, 1998, pp. 4–5.
83. The dowry system engendered feminist critique at the time as well as contemporary feminist scholarly interest. At the time, Moderata Fonte criticized the dowry system as a threat to women's virtue. She criticized the unfairness of inheritance rules that favored men and dowry regulations that constrained women, especially those women left without anything at all. These women "are forced, if they want to provide for themselves, to have recourse to those means that (as I have said) are blameworthy and despicable" Fonte (Modesta Pozzo), 1997, p. 63. As Virginia Cox explains, Venetian women's criticism of dowry and women's economic situation reached a climax just as the marriage market imposed limitations on women's ability to

marry, the usual path toward respectability and economic stability; see Cox, 1995, pp. 513–81.

84. Ruggiero, 1993, p. 30.
85. Not all Venetians believed that men were so powerless in the face of beauty and love magic. In the words of the writer Moderate Fonte, "Believe me, all that talk about magic spells is just words: men do what they do because they want to. And if you want proof, you will find men who are just as obsessed, or even more obsessed, with gambling as they are with women. So you can see what the problem is: men have vicious tendencies, to which they give too free a rein, and that's the explanation for all the crazy things they do," Fonte, 1997, p. 70.
86. Cowan, 1999, p. 277.
87. Cowan, 1999, p. 290.
88. Martini, 1986–7, pp. 305–26; Cowan, 1999, pp. 276–93.
89. Martini, 1986–7, pp. 305–26.
90. Women practiced various forms of magic to discern whether their noble lovers planned to marry them. In 1591, for example, Appollonia Colomba appeared before the Holy Office and readily confessed to having "thrown the beans" (a common form of love magic) years before in order to find out if her lover, the nobleman Vicenzo Malipiero, intended to marry her. At the time of the trial, Appollonia was married to Salvador Saonetti, who operated a furnace on the island of Murano. Nine months earlier, her name was mentioned by a former servant of the nobleman as a practitioner of magic and wife of the nobleman. ASV, Sant'Uffizio, Busta 66, fasc. Colomba, Apollonia, case begins in 1590. In another case, a woman wanted to find out if her daughter's lover intended to marry her daughter. Clara, the 70-year-old widow of a carpenter, mentioned that her daughter had been maintained by a man for three months and then wanted to find out if he intended to marry her. She therefore consulted a certain Angelica and paid her two lira for her services. ASV, Sant'Uffizio, Busta 89, fasc. Angelica, 1633.
91. Ferraro, 2001, p. 106.
92. Ferraro, 2001, pp. 107–8.
93. Sometimes the groom's family was not content with the dishonour such a bride brought to the family. See for example Eisenach, 2004, pp. 134–5.
94. "Essa si chiama Zanetta Molina per causa di quell Nobile Molina che gli levò la Verginità, per che dal med. Detto s'haverà come e qualsia il suo nome buono e vero." ASV Sant'Uffizio, Busta 114, fasc. Contra Zanettam Molini et Marietta Grimani Cipriotta, January 13, 1667.
95. On the practice of love magic, see Ruggiero, 1993, pp. 88–129.
96. ASV, Sant'Uffizio, Busta 96, fasc. Novaglia, Isabella, first booklet, fos. 45r–46v, August 7, 1640.
97. Ibid., fos. 38v-r, July 31, 1640.
98. Molho, 1988, p. 239.
99. Molho, 1979, pp. 5–33.
100. On patronage, see note 45.
101. Romano, 1987, p. 130.
102. Joanne Ferraro discusses other examples in Venice where both husband and mother-in-law offered the bride's sexual services to a gentleman and where

a father and new groom conspired to sell the sexual services of the new bride. See Ferraro, 2001, pp. 33–7.

103. Eisenach, 2004, pp. 158–9.

104. ASV Provveditori Sopra Monasteri, Busta 264, April 27, 1611, fasc. "Convertide contra Camillo Barcaruol." For more description of this case, see McGough, 1997, pp. 46–8.

105. Romano, 1996, p. xv. On the importance of master–servant relations, see also Maza, 1983 and Fairchilds, 1984.

106. Romano, 1996, pp. 77–105, 117.

107. Romano, 1996, pp. 52–3, 101–2. The Holy Office trials sometimes make reference to sexual relationships between masters and servants, although the focus of the trial itself was heretical belief. See for example Sant'Uffizio, Busta 68, fasc. De Medici, Gasparo, especially the testimony of Maria on July 18, 1591.

108. Ruggiero, 1985, p. 97. Ruggiero's evidence mostly comes from the fourteenth and fifteenth centuries. The pattern of failing to prosecute noblemen for sex crimes continued in the sixteenth and seventeenth centuries. See Walker, 1998, p. 100.

109. ASV, Sant'Uffizio, Busta 68, fasc. De Medici, Gasparo, see esp. testimony of July 30, 1591.

110. ASV, Esecutori contro la Bestemmia, Busta 61, March 4, 1627 f. 49v. See also note 57 for more literature on defloration cases.

111. The relationship between criminal prosecutions and extent of rape is not always clear, because women are often reluctant to report rapes when it is seldom prosecuted and the burden of proof is placed upon the victim, as was usually the case in Renaissance Italy. Samuel Cohn actually argues that the extent of rape in Florence probably increased during the fifteenth century because prosecution declined. See Cohn, 1996, p. 30.

112. Walker, 1998, p. 100.

113. Roussiaud, 1988, p. 21.

114. Ruggiero, 1985, p. 96. Ruggiero's study focuses on fourteenth- and fifteenth-century cases, but the broad pattern of remaining more sympathetic to victims according to age and status emerged during the sixteenth and seventeenth centuries. See also Cohn, 1996, pp. 98–136, esp. 119–20.

115. Schleiner, 1994, p. 508.

116. On Saint Disdier, see Massimo Gemin, "Le Cortigiane di Venezia e i viaggiatori stranieri," in *Il gioco dell'amore*, p. 76.

117. Wolff, 2005, pp. 417–40, esp. pp. 424, 432–3, 437.

2 The Suspected Culprits: Dangerously Beautiful Prostitutes and Debauched Men

This chapter is an expansion and revision of an earlier paper, "Purifying the Body Politic: Venice's Response to Syphilis," at The Body in Early Modern Italy Conference, Johns Hopkins University, Baltimore, MD, on October 17, 2002 and a book chapter, "Quarantining Beauty: The French Disease in Early Modern Venice," in Kevin Siena (ed.) *Sins of the Flesh: Responding to Sexual Disease in Early*

Modern Europe (Toronto: Centre for Reformation and Renaissance Studies, 2005), pp. 211–38.

1. Antonio Musa Brasavola's treatise on the French disease was published both on its own and as part of a collection in Venice. The treatise *De morbid Gallici vocati curatione* formed the final part of *Examen omnium Loch; idest linctuum, suffuf, idest pulverum, aquarum, decoctionum, oleorum, quorum apud Ferrarienses pharmacopolas usus est, ubi De morbo Gallico...* (Venice: Apud Juntas, 1553); for Musa Brasavola's contribution to the collection of various authors' works on the French disease, see *De morbo gallico omnia quae extant apud omnes medicos cujuscunque nationis....* (Venice, Jordanum Zilettum, 1566–7), pp. 564–634. The Latin treatise was also published in Lyons multiple times in 1555, 1556, and 1561. On Musa Brasavola's theory, see Foa, 1990, p. 39.

2. Rostinio, *Trattato del Mal Francese*, ff. 21r-v. The 1559 edition is a reprint of the 1556 edition. "*Nel campo de Francesi del mille quattrocento era una meretrice bellissima, la quale nella bocca della matrice haveva una apostema putrefatta, et gli huomini che usavano con lei fregolando il collo della matrice, per la humidità & putredine del loco, nel mēbro virile cōtrahevano una dispositione, che ulcerava,*" f. 21r. "*Et questo male cominciò a macular prima un'huomo, poscia due, et tre, &cēto, perche quella era publica meretrice & bellissima. & si come la natura humana è appetitosa del coito, molte donne usando con questi huomini, infettate si trovavano di tal male. Et queste l'han participato con altri huomini, tal che il detto male si è sparso per tutta la Italia, Francia, & per tutta l'Europa,*" f. 21v. From the 1553 Latin edition of *Examen omnium*, "*Scortum aderat nobilissimū ac pulcherrimū in vteri ore putrefactum gerens abscessum. Viri qui cum illa coibāt adiuuante etiam humiditate ac putredine, dum membra virilia per uteri collum perfricabāt, ob loci etiam putredinem in eor(um) virilibus membris prauam quondam affectionem contrahebant, qua exulcerabantur,*" f 194r. "*Hœc lues unum primo infecit hominem, postea duos, tres, & centum, quia illa erat publica meretrix & pulcherrima, & vt procax est humana natura in coitum, multe mulieres cum his vitiates viris coeuntes lue ista infecte sunt, quam deinde aliis viris sunt impartite, vt deniq; lues per totā Italiam sparsa sit, & per Gallias, & brevibus p(er) vniuersam Europam,*" f 194r.

3. "*Il detto male si è sparso per tutta la Italia, Francia, & per tutta l'Europa. Ho anco udito, che è in gran vigore nell'Asia, & che anco ne machiata l'Africa. Niente ragiono dell'India, che egli ivi è famigliarissimo,*" f. 21v.

4. Foa, 1990, pp. 27–8, 38–9.

5. Qualtiere and Slights argue that the development of the idea of contagion in the sixteenth century shifted the focus of ethical discourse to the individual. See Qualtiere and Slights, 2003, pp. 1–24.

6. Deanna Shemek, "'Mi mostrano a ditto tutti quanti': Disease, Deixis, and Disfiguration in the *Lamento di una cortigiana ferrarese*," in Paul Ferrara, Eugenio Giusti, and Jane Tylus (eds.) *Italiana XI: Medusa's Gaze: Essays on Gender, Literature, and Aesthetics in Honor of Robert J. Rodini*, 2004, pp. 49–64; Schleiner, 1994, pp. 499–517.

7. Literary scholars have been more successful than historians in recognizing references to diseased prostitutes as symbols of cultural anxiety. An excellent example is Deanne Shemek, 2004, pp. 49–64. See also the various essays in Siena, 2005.

8. Poirer, 2005, pp. 157–76.

9. Treichler, 1988, p. 229.

10. Shilts, 1987. For commentary on Gaetan Dugas as "Patient Zero," see Griffin, 2000 and Treichler, 1988, pp. 190–266, esp. p. 217.
11. For a similar discussion of how living people can become representatives of a particular disease, see Leavitt, 1996. Although others also suffered from typhoid fever, Mary Mallon's role as a cook, her gender, and her Irish origins all contributed to public fascination with her as a singular representative of this disease.
12. Farmer, 1992.
13. Deanna Shemek, "Mi mostrano a ditto tutti quanti";" Winfried Schleiner, "Infection and Cure through Women: Renaissance Constructions of the French Disease"; Domenico Zanrè, "French Diseases and Italian Responses: Representations of the Mal Francese in the Literature of Cinquecento Tuscany," in Siena, 2005, pp. 187–208.
14. Eamon, 1998, pp. 1–31.
15. Massa, 1566.
16. Corradi, 1871, pp. 1–32.
17. Parenti, quoted by Corradi, pp. 15–16. "Settembre 1496. Non sarà inconueniente far memoria della nuoua malattia uenuta a questi tempi, chiamata rogna franciosa, la quale in tutte parti del mondo si distese. Fava doglia intensissima; durava 8 in 10 mesi."
18. Corradi, p. 19. "*Et non vera rimedio se non lasarla fare suo corso et se trovava che le feminine lo avavano in la natura e per questo ne funo chazate molte meretrize da bologna e da ferara e altri luoghi.*"
19. Corradi, p. 19. "*e questo provene per li homini hanno a fare con donne immonde.*"
20. For a useful summary of the medical traditions regarding women's bodies, see Maclean, 1980, pp. 28–46.
21. Quoted by Sperling, 1999, p. 92. Sperling describes how the Venus-Virgin metaphor created a sense of wonder among Venice's admirers; see pp. 83–96.
22. Quoted by Eglin, 2001, pp. 11–12; see also Muir, 1981, pp. 53–4.
23. Sperling, 1999, pp. 97–8; Rosenthal, 1992, p. 9.
24. Muir, 1981, pp. 46–7.
25. Rosenthal, 1992, pp. 13–19.
26. Eglin, 2001, p. 3.
27. Wilson, 2005, pp. 117–18.
28. For the ways in which images of chaste women could evoke the images of prostitutes and vice versa because they are defined in opposition to each other in Renaissance Ferrara, see Deanna Shemek, *Ladies Errant*, pp. 38–9.
29. Steele, 1997, pp. 481–502.
30. Yavneh, 1993, pp. 133–57.
31. Yavneh, 1993, pp. 133–4.
32. Yavneh, 1993, pp. 138–9; Cropper, 1976, pp. 374–94. The best-known Renaissance treatise on women's beauty is by Agnolo Firenzuola. He constructed an ideal woman made of the various parts of women who attended a fictional party in his dialogue *On the Beauty of Women*, trans. Eisenbichler and Murray, 1992. On Firenzuola's life, see Eisenbichler and Murray, 1992, pp. xiii–xviii.
33. Rogers, 1988, pp. 47–87, on p. 56.

34. Agnolo Firenzuola, *On The Beauty of Women*, p. 14. Domenico Zanré describes Firenzuola's bout with the French disease in "French Diseases and Italian Responses: Representations of the *mal francese* in the Literature of Cinquecento Tuscany," in Siena, 2005, pp. 187–210, on pp. 200–3.

35. Brown, 2001; Ames-Lewis and Rogers, 1998; Steele, 1997, pp. 481–502.

36. Giovanni Marinello, *Gli ornamenti delle donne* (Venice: Francesco de' Franceschi Senese, 1562); on the relationship between cosmetics, beauty, and medicine, see Laughran, 2003, pp. 43–82.

37. Della Porta, 1598, p. 86. On Della Porta, see Eamon, 1994, pp. 194–233.

38. Pancino, 2003, pp. 5–42, on pp. 5, 32–4. This moralistic discourse was still evident in the early eighteenth century, when writers such as Francesco Beretta wrote advice manuals for noblemen choosing a spouse.

39. Literally, "Con le bellezze non si mangia," and "Ogni bela scarpa deventa bruta ciabata." I have translated "scarpa" as slipper to reflect the word's positive association in English (such as Cinderella's glass slippers) and translated "ciabata" as shoe to reflect the negative connotations in English of old shoe. Cited by Pancino, "Soffrire per ben comparire," pp. 36–7.

40. Rollo-Koster, 2002, pp. 109–44, on pp. 129–30.

41. On the iconography of Mary Magdalene, see Mosco, 1986; Haskins, 1993; and Malvern, 1975. On the sexualization of touch represented visually in Renaissance art, see 1993, pp. 198–224.

42. Quotation from Findlen, 1993, pp. 49–108, on pp. 64–5. On the eroticism of Renaissance art, especially Titian's Venus of Urbino, see Freedberg, 1989, esp. p. 17.

43. Goffen, 1997, pp. 1–5, 179–80.

44. Lewis Wager's 1566 play about Mary Magdalene, for example, can be seen as a critique of Catholic mores. See Badir, 1999, pp. 1–20.

45. Cameron, 1991, pp. 79–81; Fitzgerald, 1988; Lualdi and Thayer, 2000.

46. Arrizabalaga et al., 1997, pp. 56–87.

47. Montrose, 1991, pp. 4–5.

48. Campbell, 1992, p. 9.

49. Eatough, 1984, p. 87.

50. Eatough, 1984, p. 93.

51. The presence of Girolamo Fracastoro's name on this list may surprise a few readers who associate him with refuting the idea of the French disease's New World origins in his epic poem *De Syphilis*, credited with providing the name for the disease. Nonetheless, Fracastoro's narrative strategies reinforced the association between disease, the New World, and the female body. See Campbell, 1992, pp. 20–2.

52. Horodowich, 2005, pp. 1031–62.

53. Deanna Shemek, "Mi mostrano a ditto tutti quanti," pp. 51–3.

54. Deanna Shemek, "Mi mostrano a ditto tutti quanti," pp. 55–7; Domenico Zanrè, "French Diseases and Italian Responses," pp. 189–91.

55. Rosenthal, 1992, pp. 44–5.

56. Rosenthal, 1992, pp. 165–6. Rosenthal's translation of "quell ache mantien guerra/Contro la sanità. Mare del morbo."

57. Henry III's critics alleged that he contracted a venereal disease during this visit, another example of how disease served as a symbol of moral disorder and could be used to shame or discredit people. Poirier, 2005, p. 170.

58. Schuler, 1991, pp. 209–22. Rona Goffen wisely points out that the actual identity of Titian's models is comparatively unimportant to understanding his paintings, in which "the anonymous becomes a mythic being, she becomes Sacred and Profane Love or Venus herself, or indeed she becomes the very embodiment of beauty. And in this process, her historical identity is taken from her: her own biography is irrelevant," Goffen, 1997, p. 149.

59. One of the most widely circulated guidebooks was Coryat, 1611, in which he described his visit to a courtesan's house. He justified his visit on the grounds that he tried to convert the courtesan to religious life, but was unsuccessful. Besides, his observation of vice would only consolidate his commitment to leading a virtuous life. "For I think that a virtuous man will be the more confirmed and settled in vertue by the observation of some vices, then if he did not at all know what they were," p. 271.

60. Karras, 1996, pp. 32, 138.

61. Pavan, October–December 1980, p. 242.

62. Pavan, October–December 1980, pp. 241–88.

63. As Leah Lydia Otis argues in the case of Languedoc, the change in attitude toward prostitution was part of a "desire for change in sexual morality [that] had been growing since the late Middle Ages," Otis, 1985, pp. 43–5. In Augsburg, after the public brothel closed in 1532, prostitutes depended on fewer numbers of clients in longer-term relationships. "The boundary between prostitute and non-prostitute became blurred. No longer a group of dishonorable women, clearly defined by where they lived and what they wore, there was little difference between prostitutes, fornicators or adulteresses—indeed, any woman might be a prostitute." Roper, "Discipline and Respectability: Prostitution and the Reformation in Augsburg," *History Workshop Journal*, p. 21. For France, see Rossiaud, 1988.

64. Rosenthal, 1992, pp. 102–10, 11; Ruggiero, 1985, p. 162.

65. Coryat, 1611, p. 264.

66. Chojnacka, 2001, pp. 22–3.

67. Gemin, 1990, pp. 46–53.

68. On the importance of Venice to English debates about political liberty, see Muir, 1981, pp. 51–5.

69. Coryat's narrative makes frequent reference to the hypocrisy of Venetian institutions: the friar who allegedly had sexual relations with 99 nuns, an orphanage which existed so that courtesans could more easily abandon their children, the existence of a convent for retired prostitutes, etc. See Coryat, 1611, pp. 253, 269, 268.

70. Coryat, 1611, p. 265. Margaret Rosenthal's discussion of traveler's accounts of Venetian courtesans as a literary theme is especially effective. See Rosenthal, 1992, pp. 11–14, 19–24.

71. Coryat, 1611, p. 271.

72. Healy, 2001, pp. 130, 142–3, 152.

73. Cohen, 1998, pp. 392–409.

74. Deanne Shemek, "Mi mostrano a ditto tutti quanti," pp. 57–60.

75. Ascanio Centorio, *Discorsi di Guerra* (Venice: Gabriel Giolito de' Ferrari, 1567), f. 12v. "Scipio Africano in Ispagna, essendogli presentata una bellissima giovane avanti, non solo da quella si astenne, ma non volse pur mirarla, et commesse che fosse restituita a suoi parenti."

76. For example, Domenico Mora criticized the general indiscipline of soldiers, including such faults as killing out of caprice and "forcing women" (*chi sforzerà donne*). Mora, 1569, f. 8r. See also Hanlon, 1998, esp. p. 265.
77. Centorio, *Discorsi di guerra*, ff. 57v, 39v.
78. Gallucci, 2003, pp. 138–41.
79. For a detailed study of the Interdict controversy, see Bouwsma, 1968, pp. 339–482.
80. Muir, 2007, pp. 61–108.
81. Muir, 2007, pp. 61–108.
82. The conflict between libertines and moralists made use of the trope of the diseased body in seventeenth-century France as well. One libertine poet ended his "lament" for having contracted the disease from intercourse with a woman by not renouncing sex (as was typical of the moralistic genre) but by vowing to have only anal sex in the future if he survived. "God I truly repent for a life so untrue:/ And if right away I am not killed by your wrath, I vow hereafter to screw only in the ass," quoted by Poirer, 2005, p. 173.
83. So-called obscene literature, such as the writings of Pietro Aretino, were first prohibited by Pope Paul IV's Index of Prohibited Books in 1559. Although Venetian booksellers protested the Index, the papacy responded with economic reprisals against Venetian booksellers that ultimately proved successful. See Grendler, 1977, pp. 116–22.
84. Schleiner, 1994.
85. Maclean, 1999, pp. 127–55, on pp. 133 and 140.
86. Schleiner, 1994, pp. 499–517, on p. 504.
87. Foa, 1990, p. 39. In addition, Pietro Andrea Mattioli also wrote about intercourse with leprous women but provided no details.
88. Foa, 1990, p. 40.
89. Daston and Park, 2001, p. 145; on Paracelsus' relationship to natural and preternatural philosophy, p. 160; on monsters, pp. 173–214.
90. Porter, 1997, p. 205.
91. Daston and Park 2001, p. 200.
92. Porter, 1997, p. 182.
93. Schleiner, 1994, pp. 389–410, on p. 399.
94. On Lippi's and Christus's portraits of women, see Brown et al., 2001, pp. 106–7, 138–9.
95. Estienne, 1546, pp. 294, 300, 310, 312; the pastoral scene is on p. 312 and the woman reclining with legs splayed is on p. 310. On the association between Estienne and Italian erotic images, see Carlino, 1999, pp. 23–6. A few of Titian's images have strongly muscled women, such as the 1560 painting *Mars, Venus, and Amor*, as do the erotic images in *I Modi* described in note 93.
96. Giulio Romano drew a series of these images which were accompanied by Pietro Aretino's text. They were first published in 1524 and reappeared in woodcut edition in Venice in 1550. See Lawner, 1989.
97. Foa, 1990, p. 40.
98. The 1559 edition, for example, states that Rostinio has translated parts of Brasavola's work and added his own work. The 1565 edition makes no mention of Brasavola, but makes references to the popular empiric Leonardo

Fioravanti's book *Capriccio Medicinale* (9v), a reference that did not appear in the 1559 edition.
99. Eamon, 1994, pp. 168–82.
100. Eamon, 1994, pp. 10–16.
101. Rostinio, 1565, p. f. 9v.
102. Daston and Park, 2001, p. 200; see also Paré, 1982, chapter 20. "An Example of the Mixture or Mingling of Seed," p. 67. "There are monsters that are born with a form that is half-animal and the other [half] human, or retaining everything [about them] from animals, which are produced by sodomists and atheists who 'join together' and break out of their bounds—unnaturally—with animals, and from this are born several hideous monsters that bring great shame to those who look at them or speak of them."
103. Nutton, 1983, pp. 27–8.
104. Arrizabalaga, 1994, pp. 260–3.
105. Palmer, 1978, pp. 91–3, and Nutton, 1983, pp. 1–34. In practice, public health officials recognized the possibility of contagion by imposing quarantine not only on sick individuals, but also on those who had been in contact with the sick. Carmichael, 1991, pp. 213–56.
106. Allen, 2000, p. 34.
107. Qualtiere and Slights, 2003, pp. 16–18.
108. Leoniceno had earlier argued that the French disease struck first in the genitals not because of sexual transmission, but because these parts were more susceptible to putrefaction due to their natural humidity and heat. Other commentators, such as Almenar, rejected this idea on the grounds that all diseases should then begin in the genitals. See Arrizabalaga, 2005, p. 43.
109. "Se dimãdi in questo male, che cosa sia questa venenosita, dicemo, che è una mala dispositione senza nome, ne da niuno è definita dico ma la dispositione di questo male qual è nasciuto, & dalla mala qualita dell'aere, & dalla frictione nel cavernoso loco della donna, dove è mala dispositione il male è da numerar tra li contagiosi," (f. 21v).
110. Rostinio's complete explanation of these mechanisms is the following: "Nel campo de Francesi del mille quattrocento era una meretrice bellissima, la quale nella bocca della matrice haveva una apostema putrefatta, et gli huomini che usavano con lei fregolando il collo della matrice, per la humidità & putredine del loco, nel mẽbro virile cõtrahevano una dispositione, che ulcerava, & per il mẽbro qual'è mollissimo ascẽdeva una mala qualita fino alle vie emũtorie, & alle parti del l'inguini. Et la natura per scacciar fuori la mala qualita venenosa ivi facea tumori, et ivi trasmettera la materia. Poi quella mala qualita fino al figato ascẽdeva, & maculava il sangue," f. 21r.
111. Arrizabalaga, 2005, p. 44.

3 Stigma Reinforced: The Problem of Incurable Cases of a Curable Disease

Part of this chapter is revised and expanded from an earlier article. See Laura J. McGough, "Demons, Nature or God? Witchcraft Accusations and the French Disease in Early Modern Venice," *Bulletin of the History of Medicine* Vol. 80: 2 (Summer 2006), 219–46.

1. Arrizabalaga et al., 1997, pp. 29, 131–5.
2. Arrizabalaga et al., 1997, pp. 56–87.
3. French and Arrizabalaga, 1998, pp. 248–87, on pp. 254–6.
4. French and Arrizabalaga, 1998, pp. 257–8.
5. Arrizabalaga et al., 1997, pp. 100–3, 139–42. On other treatment such as the dry stove, see pp. 137–9.
6. Arrizabalaga et al., 1997, pp. 266–7.
7. Siraisi, 1997; on Cardano's alleged cure for a disease known as phthisis and its comparison to the French disease, see p. 24; on reasons why the French disease was seen as curable, see p. 34.
8. Siena, 2004, p. 81.
9. Aretino, 1976, p. 222. Letter of August 22, 1542. Aretino's work is certainly more complex than simple pornography or even eroticism. He intended to criticize what he regarded as an excessively abstract academic culture and wanted to emphasize the importance of concrete, material reality. At the same time, he also wanted to examine the different "motors" of human life, which he saw as money and sex. Whereas men were often equally driven by both, some women, especially prostitutes, were only driven by money, and were therefore not caught between these two often conflicting forces. See Larivaille, 1980, esp. pp. 99–100, 172–3.
10. Arrizabalaga, 2005, p. 41.
11. Arrizabalaga, 2005, p. 35.
12. Arrizabalaga, 2005, pp. 33–55, on pp. 47–8.
13. Arrizabalaga, 2005, p. 49.
14. Winfried Schleiner, "Moral Attitudes toward Syphilis and Its Prevention in the Renaissance," *Bulletin of the History of Medicine* 68 (1994), 389–410, on 398–400.
15. ASV, Giustizia Vecchia, Busta 74, Reg. 95, August 2, 1633 f. 1r, August 9, 1633 f. 2v. Thanks to James Shaw for showing me this case.
16. Siena, 2004, pp. 1–61.
17. Trivellato, 1998, pp. 47–82.
18. The groundbreaking work on stigma is Goffman, 1963. More recent work has emphasized how the development of stigma is embedded in broader power inequalities in society. See Parker and Aggleton, 2003, pp. 15–24; Link and Phelan, 2001, pp. 363–85.
19. Goffman, 1963, pp. 3–4.
20. On books of secrets, see Eamon, 1994.
21. Massa, 1566, p. iii. The same was true in seventeenth-century London, where medical advertisements for the French disease were common, and female healers treated women who were too ashamed to consult with male doctors. See Siena, 2001, pp. 199–224.
22. See Mercurio, 1621, p. 280. On Mercurio's place in the history of Italian obstetrics, see Pancino, 1984, p. 27. Interestingly, Giovanni Marinello's book "for chaste and young women" did not include recipes for French disease sores, again suggesting that the disease brought some shame for unmarried women. His book does include recipes for hiding marks due to smallpox, for example, and the various illnesses which can do damage to a woman's external beauty. Marinello, 1574, see esp. f. 1v; for smallpox, third book, chapter X, f. 204r.

23. Porter, 2000, p. 132.
24. Cortese, 1588, pp. 13–16. On books of secrets, see Eamon, 1994. Little is known about Isabella Cortese's life, although Eamon surmises that she must have been of high social status because of her literacy. She was the only female author of a book of secrets, an extremely popular genre in the sixteenth and seventeenth centuries. On Cortese, see Eamon, 1994, p. 137.
25. Siena, 2004, pp. 30–61.
26. *Opera Nuova Intitolata Dificio di Ricette, nella quale si contengono tre utilissimi ricettari* (Venice, 1526), f. 19v; *Opera Nova Intitolata Dificio de Recette nella quale si contengono tre utilissimi recettari,* (Venice, 1530), f. 17r.
27. *Secreti Diversi & miracolosi,* (Venice: Alessandro Gardano, 1578), pp. 28–43.
28. Guaiacum was a wood from the West Indies widely used as a cure for the French disease. The wood was supposed to be ground to sawdust, then soaked in water in a ratio of eights parts water to one part wood. The water should then be boiled until reduced to half its original volume; the foam produced during boiling should be dried and used as a medicine. See Arrizabalaga et al., 1997, pp. 100 2.
29. *Secreti Diversi & miracolosi,* (Venice: Alessandro Gardano, 1578), p. 43.
30. Henderson, 2006, pp. 303, 317.
31. Palmer, 1985, pp. 100–17, on p. 101–2. One apothecary noted his happiness at receiving roots of a plant named *colchicum syriacum alexandrinum* (a flowering plant in the lily family) from a surgeon in the Venetian fleet; roots of this plant were added to guaiacum for treatment of the French disease.
32. Palmer, 1985, p. 105.
33. David Gentilcore, "Charlatans, The Regulated Marketplace and the Treatment of Venereal Disease in Italy," in Kevin Siena (ed.), *Sins of the Flesh*, pp. 57–80, on p. 73.
34. Siena, 2001, pp. 199–224.
35. Pomata, 1998, p. 92; Gentilcore, 2005, p. 70.
36. Gentilcore, 2005, p. 69.
37. ASV Prov. alla Sanità, Busta 736, January 8, 1590 m.v., Feb. 15, 1590 m.v., undated application for *mal* francese ff. 50r-51r, June 19, 1595; Busta 737, July 14, 1597, February 3, 1600 m.v., March 14, 1602, April 18, 1603, July 8, 1603, July 30, 1603, August 8, 1603, March 5, 1607. On the Sanità and secret recipes, see Laughran, 1998, p. 170 n.123. The Sanità also advised the College of Physicans about a secret powder said to be miraculous in the cure of the French disease in 1579. See Palmer, 1983, p.11 n. 38.
38. ASV Prov. alla Sanità, Busta 736, undated application for *mal francese* ff. 50r-51r.
39. In fact, venereal disease remedies account for only an average of 2.6 percent of all licensed remedies in select Italian cities between 1550 and 1800. This percentage does not describe sales volume, however. See Gentilcore, 2005, p. 73.
40. Prov. alla Sanità, Busta 737, March 14, 1602.
41. Prov. alla Sanità, Busta 737, April 18, 1603, f. 139r-v. The Health Board approved this request on April 19.
42. Gentilcore, 1998, p. 23.
43. ASV, Sant'Uffizio, Busta 95, fasc. Refiletti Angela, Margherita Bergamo, test. of Olivia widow of Battista, August 17, 1638. "Dicevano che andava in barca,

et che vestita tutta di seta, et che andava con gran pompa, per quanto mi diceva mi fia."

44. See also the description of the Italian charlatan Jacopo Coppa, "standing on a rich carpet, holding a golden scepter, dressed, in the fashion of the Medici, in a tunic of black velvet over a long skirt of the same material." Gambacini, 2004, p. 85. Charlatans and mountebanks were well-known for their costume and fine clothing, especially for wearing velvet and gold. Male charlatans often dressed in "exotic oriental clothes" typical of Turks, or as physicians. Despite sumptuary laws to limit this practice, charlatans continued to wear these clothes. See Katritzky, 2001, pp. 121–253, esp. pp. 140–2.

45. ASV, Sant'Uffizio, Busta 95, fasc. Refiletti Angela, Margherita Bergamo, testimony of Angela Refiletti, September 16, 1638.

46. ASV, Sant'Uffizio, Busta 95, fasc. Refiletti Angela, Margherita Bergamo, testimony of Jo.es Bazizer Bergomer, 34 years old, August 16, 1638.

47. ASV, Sant'Uffizio, Busta 66, fasc. Orsetta Padova, testimony of Orsetta, May 24, 1590. "Io vivo delle mie fatiche et de mei sudori, che medico gentilhomini, et Mons.ri et hora medico un prete da Muran che ha nome pre Paulo, il qual ha un'ulcera nel membro."

48. She was sentenced on July 7, 1590 and forbidden to practice medicine again.

49. There is no evidence that women in particular specialized in French disease cures. Female healers often specialized in women's illnesses, especially related to retention of menstruation. See Pomata, 1999, pp. 119–43, esp. p. 129.

50. ASV, Sant'Uffizio, Busta 70, fasc. Maddalena Greca et Ottavio de Rossi, testimony of June 2, 1615 and July 30, 1615.

51. Menghi, 1605; original edition 1576. "Il che per dar ad intendere al volgo, & cavarne danari, fingono questi Malefici d'applicargli certi remedi naturali, quale niente giouana se non per coprire le loro sceleratezze," p. 230.

52. ASV Sant'Uffizio, Busta 30, fasc. 31 Helen La Draga, testimony of August 14, 1571.

53. ASV, Sant'Uffizio, Busta 97, Fasc. Compiliti, Giovanna, testimony of September 10, 1641.

54. One of the best descriptions of the variety of healing practices is Gentilcore, 1998.

55. Laurence Brockliss and Colin Jones, 1997, *The Medical World of Early Modern France*, p. 633; Margaret Pelling, *Medical Conflicts in Early Modern London*, pp. 262, 340. Pelling points out that surgeons and irregular practitioners rather than physicians provided much of the pox treatment in London. On the lack of moralizing by Italian physicians and surgeons, see Schleiner, 1994, pp. 389–410, on pp. 397–8 and Gentilcore, 2005, pp. 57–80, on pp. 59–60.

56. On Falloppio and Rudio, see Schleiner, 1994, pp. 399–404; on Morgagni, see Gentilcore, 2005, p. 61. On discomfort with same-sex sexual relations, see Berco, 2007, pp. 92–113.

57. Gentilcore, 2005, p. 59.

58. Rostinio, 1565, p. 26. "*Se alcuno ha usato con puttane, & che gli venga caroli in bocca, & che nelle fauci, nella gola venga ulceratione… ne facilmente si puo curare, ma par che vada via, poscia ritnorni, costui ha mal francese.*"

59. Stein, 2006, pp. 617–47, on p. 638.

60. Stein, 2006, pp. 617–9.

61. Rostinio, *Trattato del Mal Francese* (1565), 26.

62. Siena, 2007, pp. 92–113.

63. For the case of Bologna see, Pomata, 1998.
64. ASV, Giustizia Vecchia, Busta 74, Reg. 94, December 3, 1624, December 4, 1624, December 11, 1624, March 5, 1625, April 28, 1625. Thanks to James Shaw for pointing out this case to me.
65. Pomata, 1998, p. 97.
66. McGough, 2006, pp. 219–46.
67. Eamon, 1994, pp. 259–66.
68. Mercurio, 1658, p. 310. "quasi ciascuno per ogni mal di testa, e per qualunque altra infermità, prima va à ritrovar la malefica, ò strega, che la Segni, e poi il Medico, e per mal di madre, per febre terzane, ò quartane, per piaghe, e sluogamenti, e infino per il mal francese si fanno segnar da queste veramente streghe." On Mercurio, see Tedeschi, 1991, pp. 234, 239; Gentilcore, 1998, pp. 59, 80–1; Eamon, 1994, pp. 190, 261–2.
69. Mercurio, 1658, p. 15.
70. Mercurio, 1658, pp. 51, 67. Mercurio recommended purgatives for the French disease.
71. Mercurio, 1658, p. 194.
72. Mercurio, 1658, p. 313. To remove women from "the world" usually meant to remove them from worldly life in order to adopt a religious life.
73. On exorcism and healing, see O'Neil, 1984, pp. 53–83.
74. Ruggiero, 2001.
75. It is unclear whether Sarpi's codification of laws would have resulted in greater administrative attention to recording and preserving trial records, greater confidence in pursuing these cases, or greater assertiveness by the Venetian Inquisition in asserting its prerogatives. See Schutte, 2001, pp. 33–4, 97.
76. Martin, 1989, pp. 76–8.
77. Martin, 1989, p. 226.
78. Monter, 1976, pp. 23–4. On this issue throughout Europe, see Levack, 1995, pp. 133–41.
79. Martin, 1989, p. 226.
80. For an illuminating discussion of the relationship between social relations, illness, and witchcraft in South Africa, see Ashforth, 2000.
81. Briggs, *Witches and Neighbors*, p. 75.
82. Martin, 1993, pp. 49–70.
83. Martin, 1993, p. 236.
84. Tedeschi, 1991, pp. 134–5; Monter, 1990. For a useful introduction to the geographical variations in witch trials and witch-hunts, see Levack, 1995. A fine study of the procedures of a witchcraft trial outside the jurisdiction of the Inquisition is Kunze, 1987.
85. The best recent description of the workings of the Venetian inquisition is by Schutte, 2001, pp. 26–41.
86. Tedeschi, 1991, p. 235.
87. Tedeschi, 1991, p. 234; O'Neil, 1987, p. 97.
88. Schutte, 2001, p. 40.
89. Martin, 1989, p. 189; Marietta Colonna was found guilty of suspected heresy and punished but not executed; see pp. 186–8.
90. ASV, Sant'Uffizio, Busta 79, fasc. Savioni, Camilla. Denunciation made by Girolamo Marcello on February 21, 1624 includes the accusations against Camilla.
91. ASV, Sant'Uffizio, Busta 79, fasc. Savioni, Camilla.

92. Ruggiero, 1993, pp. 24–56.
93. Weaver, 2003, pp. 126–53, on pp. 131–2. Evidence that this epic was known outside of literary elites appears in Inquisition trials; see Guido Ruggiero, 1993, p. 44.
94. The most famous example is the character of Alcida who ensnared the hero Ruggiero by means of bewitchment in Ariosto's *Orlando Furioso*. See Kisacky, 2000, p. 106. An exception to the story of the typical "Renaissance enchantress" is found in Torquato Taso's *Il Rinaldo*, in which the character Floriana seduces not through magic but through "her great beauty, her courtesy, and her other virtues." See Cavallo, 2004, p. 178.
95. MacDonald, *Mystical Bedlam*, p. 210.
96. ASV, Sant'Uffizio, Busta 79, fasc. Savioni, Camilla, testimony of August 17, 1624. "Io non giurarei che il suo male non procedesse anco da male sopranaturale, perche il diavolo pot. decipere et. medicos."
97. ASV, Sant'Uffizio, Busta 79, fasc. Savioni, Camilla, testimony of August 17, 1624. "Et vedendo moi la pertinaccia dei mali et la varietà di essi, et alcuno anco straord.rio et non frequente, alcuni anco medici entrono in che vi potesse esser qualche lesion de fatture, ma però non vi erano segni dimostrativi."
98. O'Neil, 1984, p. 54.
99. ASV, Sant'Uffizio, Busta 79, fasc. Savioni, Camilla, testimony of May 9, 1624.
100. On the Soccorso, see Rosenthal, 1992, pp. 131–2; Pullan, 1971.
101. ASV, Sant'Uffizio, Busta 79, fasc. Savioni, Camilla, testimony of February 24, 1624.
102. Ibid., testimony of March 1. On love magic, see Ruggiero, 1993, esp. pp. 107–29.
103. Andrea's relationships with other women had been mentioned earlier in the trial. ASV, Sant'Uffizio, Busta 79, fasc. Savioni, Camilla, testimony of March 1, 1624.
104. ASV, Sant'Uffizio, Busta 79, fasc. Savioni, Camilla, testimony of July 27, 1624.
105. ASV, Provveditori alla Sanità, Necrologio Reg. 853, year 1624, September 29, 1624.
106. Bylebyl, 1993, pp. 52, 59–60.
107. Bylebyl, 1993, p. 49.
108. In Venice, women of all ages were denounced for witchcraft, although the popular stereotype often focused on older women. For the age breakdown of those denounced of witchcraft in Venice, see Martin, 1989, p. 228. Throughout Europe as a whole, however, women over the age of 50 were the most common targets, partly because of fears expressed in the stereotype of the "sexually voracious old hag." See Levack, 1995, pp. 141–5.
109. ASV, records of the Holy Office (Sant'Uffizio), Busta 77, fasc. 21, contra Bellina Loredana, 1624. See also Ruggiero, 1993, pp. 116–7.
110. ASV, Sant'Uffizio, Busta 77, fasc. 21, contra Bellina Loredana, December 10, 1624.
111. ASV, Sant'Uffizio, Busta 72, fasc. Domeniga cameriera della Signora Margarita.
112. Quoted by Ruggiero, 2001, p. 12.
113. Quoted by Ruggiero, 2001, p. 37.
114. Ruggiero, 2001, p. 41.

115. Ruggiero, 2001, p. 40.
116. Martin, 1989, pp. 200–1.
117. Martin, 1989, p. 201.
118. Harley, "Mental Illness, Magical Medicine and the Devil," p. 143.
119. Ferraro, 2001, pp. 126–7.
120. ASV Guidice Petizion, Terminazioni, reg. 133, November 18, 1616, f. 154. Thanks to Chiara Vazzoler for pointing out this case to me. See also Chiara Vazzoler, "Governare come Padri: La tutela dei Minori à Venezia (secoli XVI–XVII)" (Tesi di Laurea, University of Venice, 1996–7), pp. 30–1.
121. ASV Sant'Uffizio, Busta 98, fasc. Mattea Lavandria, May 8, 1642–August 12, 1642.
122. Briggs, *Witches and Neighbors*, p. 72.
123. Gevitz, "The Devil Hath Laughed at the Physicians," pp. 16, 24.
124. Norman Gevitz, "The Devil Hath Laughed at the Physicians," pp. 15–16.
125. Ashforth, 2002, pp. 121–43.

4   Gender and Institutions: Hospitals and Female Asylums

Part of this chapter has been revised and expanded from an earlier article. See Laura J. McGough, "Women, Private Property, and the Limitations of State Authority in Early Modern Venice," *Journal of Women's History*, Volume 14, number 3 (November 2002), 32–52.

1. Arrizabalaga et al., 1997, p. 33.
2. Henderson, 2006, p. 101.
3. ASV, Records of the Health Office (Prov. all Sanità), Busta 2, fol. 31r, February 12, 1521.
4. Palmer, 1999, pp. 87–101, on p. 93.
5. Palmer, 1999, p. 94.
6. Arrizabalaga et al., 1997, p. 183.
7. Nordio, 1996, p. 170.
8. Palmer, 1999, p. 95.
9. Nordio, 1996, p. 171.
10. de Renzi, 1999, pp. 102–31, on pp. 116–7.
11. Arrizabalaga et al., 1997, p. 190.
12. Zanré, 2005, pp. 187–208, on pp. 200–2. On how Cellini used the French disease to establish his own masculinity (evidence of his sexual conquests), see Gallucci, 2003, p. 141; on the beautiful young servant girl, p. 38.
13. Arrizabalga et al., 1997, p. 193, p. 187; ASV, Ospitali et Luoghi Pii, Diversi, Busta 1031, Notatorio, f. 78r, f. 116r.
14. Hospital governors were unsympathetic to female patients in London. See Siena, 2004, pp. 111–6.
15. ASV, Proved. alla Sanità, Busta numbers 814–23, 834–41, 850–4, 867–70. It is possible that differential mortality rates between hospitals reflected the kinds of patients they cared for, although Brian Pullan argues that both these hospitals had become "general hospitals" by the late sixteenth century. See Pullan, 1971, pp. 257, 262.

16. ASV Proved. alla Sanità, Busta 854, deaths on April 4, 1625 and April 6, 1625. Both of their ages are listed as 30 and no family members' names are included.

17. ASV Proved. alla Sanità, Busta 867, April 18, 1636 and Busta 853, April 11 and 12, 1624.

18. The years for which I compiled deaths in the Incurables hospital are 1619, 1621, 1623–5, 1636–8. ASV, Proved. alla Sanità, Busta numbers 850–4, 867–9.

19. ASV Prov. sopra Ospitali, Busta 76, "Ammalati," December 13, 1794.

20. Pullan, 1971, p. 375.

21. ASV Prov. sopra Ospitali, Busta 76, "Ammalati," October 31, 1793.

22. ASV, Prov. alla Sanità, Busta 738, 19 No. 1611, f. 32r.

23. Henderson, 2006, pp. 56–86, on p. 57.

24. Nordio, 1996, pp. 165–6. On the religious origins of the Incurables hospitals throughout Italy, see Arrizabalaga et al., 1997, chapter 8.

25. Nordio, 1996, p. 171.

26. Pullan, 1971, pp. 402–3.

27. Pullan, 1971, p. 421.

28. ASV, Sant'Uffizio, Busta 85, fasc. Mezzavillani Pietro, July 29, 1627.

29. "Sound the trumpet/I want War/I want to arm myself/Against myself ... I want War against myself/The grief that assails me/I challenge in battle/Cover me with hairshirts/O, wound me with thorns/Thus I will fight to the grave/Sound the trumpet." *La Maddalena Penitente, Oratorio in Musica da recitarsi nell'Hospitale degl'Incurabili il giorno della Santa*, dedicated to doge Alvise Contarini (Venice, 1670), f. 5r-6.

30. Cohen, 1992, p. 79.

31. van Deusen, 2001, p. xii.

32. Nordio, 1994, esp. pp. 11–17. On the religious background of the hospital's founders and of charitable works in Venice during this period, see Palmer, 1999, pp. 87–101. On the Company of Divine Love in Venice, see Tramontin, 1972, pp. 111–36.

33. Ruggerio, 1993, pp. 10–30, on pp. 26–7.

34. Rollo-Koster, 2002, pp. 109–44, esp. pp. 116–8.

35. Pullan, 1971, pp. 377–8.

36. van Deusen, 2001, pp. 137–40, 163–6.

37. Coates, 2001, p. 139.

38. *Capitoli et Ordini per il buon Governo della Congregatione del Monastero di S. Maria Maddalena delle Convertite della Giudecca* (Venice: Lovisa, 1719), pp. 8–11.

39. ASVatican, SC, E & R, Positiones, 1606 Lett. T-V, undated letter from the Convertite in Venice. "perche la predetta D.a Isabetta è giovane et è bella, desiderando benche separate dal Marito vivere honestam., et per fuggir l'occasioni dessidera Monacarsi nel Monasterio delle Convertite di Venetia."

40. Sansovino, 1581, p. 91b.

41. Pullan, 1971, p. 378.

42. Molmenti, 1906, pp. 589–90.

43. MCC Codice Cicogna 3239, November 10, 1561.

44. ASV, PS M, Busta 267, November 28, 1624; Busta 260, July 2, 1619.

45. ASV, PSM, Busta 267, August 1, 1626.

46. Archivio IRE, ZIT A1, "Costituzione e Regole della Casa delle Citelle di Venezia," Venice, 1738. Benedetto Palmio described himself as solely responsible for the selection of the Zitelle's site, but several noblewomen were also involved. See Chase, 2002, p. 73.

47. Archivio IRE, ZIT A1, "Costituzione e Regole della Casa delle Citelle di Venezia," Parte IV, Cap. III; on interviewing the girls, see Monica Chojnacka, "Charity and Poverty in Counter-Reformation Venice," paper presented at Circolo Britanico, Venice, December 1995.

48. Ciammitti, 1979, p. 469.

49. Firenzuola, *On the Beauty of Women*, pp. 63–5.

50. Chojnacka, 1998, pp. 68–91, on pp. 73–9.

51. Archivio IRE, ZIT A1, *Costituzioni e Regole della Casa delle Citelle di Venezia*, Parte Quarta, Cap. III and Cap. XV.

52. Chojnacka, 1998, pp. 73–9.

53. Douglas, 1966.

54. Carlin, 2005, p. vii.

55. Frelick, 2005, pp. 47–62.

56. Martin, 1993, p. ix.

57. Gilman, 1993, pp. 198–272, esp. pp. 201–6 on Bronzino and Titian.

58. Malvern, 1975, p. 19.

59. Boschini, 1664, p. 404; these paintings were still found at the convent at the time of its suppression under French rule, see ASV, Edwards, Busta 2, July 6, 1807. On Benfatto and Palma Giovane, see Haskins, 1993, p. 288; on del Friso, see Pallucchini, 1981, p. 22. Art within the church rather than the hallways and refectory would have been seen less often by the nuns, since they spent most of their time outside of the church and were confined to certain areas within the church. Minor artwork, such as small paintings of the Magdalene by an unknown artist, would likely have escaped the attention of contemporary observers; a few of these items appear in wills left by nuns, who bequeathed their portraits of Mary Magdalene to other nuns. See McGough, 1997, p. 127.

60. All of the following compilations of laws regarding "prostitutes" (*meretrici*) are available at the Biblioteca Marciana, Venice. *Parte presa nell'Eccellentissimo Conseglio di Pregadi sopra il vestire, & ornamenti di casa delle Meretrici*, February 21, 1542; *Parte Prese nell'Eccel.mo Conseglio di Dieci in material delle Publiche Meretrici, con l'obbligo de Barcaruoli, e Carrozzieri*, June 30 and July 8, 1615; *Terminatione Degl'Illustrissimi Sig. Provveditori alla Sanità in material de Meretrici*, December 20, 1628.

61. Laughran, 1998; and ASV, Provveditori alla Sanità, Busta 2, September 12 and 16, 1539.

62. Chase, 2002, p. 77.

63. On the history of the Giudecca, see Basaldella, 1986.

64. Palmer, 1975 and Preto, 1978. On responses to plague throughout Italy, see Cipolla, 1981 and 1976.

65. Laughran, 1998.

66. McGough, 1997, p. 132 no. 64.

67. On the impact of strict cloister in Venice, see Sperling, 1999, pp. 170–205. On cloister's impact throughout Europe, see Raimondo Creytens, "La riforma dei monastery femminili dopo i decreti tridentini," in *Concilio di Trento e la riforma tridentina*, vol. 1 Atti del convegno storico internazionale (Rome: Herder,

1965), 45–84; Ruth Liebowitz, "Virgins in the Service of Christ: The Dispute over an Active Apostolate for Women during the Counter-Reformation," in Ruether and McLaughlin, 1979, pp. 132–52.

68. "Parte Pertinente al Povero Hospedal della Pietà et delle Convertide," in *Parti prese in Consiglio Xm in Pregadi* Vol. II (Turin: Carlo Clausen, 1898), ff. 527v-529r.

69. ASPV, Archivio Segreto, Visite Pastorali a Monasteri Femminili, Busta 3 (Priuli), January 11, 1593, f. 77r-84r; Laura McGough, "'Raised from the Devil's Jaws," 1.

70. These data were compiled from ASV Convertite, Busta 1, Fasc. D. A total of 104 women entered the convent between 1656 and 1675. For more discussion of the term "raised from the devil's jaws," see McGough, 1997, p. 67.

71. ASV Convertite, Busta 1, fasc. D.

72. ASV Convertite, Busta 50, Capitoli, ff. 16–17.

73. Data compiled from ASV Convertite, Busta 1, Fasc. D. For more on these data, see McGough, 1997, pp. 70–3.

74. ASVaticano, Sacra Congregatione, Episcoporum et Regularium, Positiones, Lett. S-V, July 24, 1600, Venice.

75. Ruggiero, 1985, pp. 41–2; Cohen, 1988, pp. 21–30.

76. ASVaticano, Sacra Congregatione, Episcoporum et Regularium, Positiones, September–November 1676, f. November 20, 1676, Padua.

77. Rape victims represented a minority of women in the Convertite, but their presence was persistent. Seven-year old Gratoisa Vettoni, for example, entered the Convertite after having been raped by Olivo Jurlini in 1659. See ASV, Esecutori contro la Bestemmia, Busta 62, Raspe, January 24, 1658 m.v., f. 23r. Court records survive for only a portion of the seventeenth century, so a complete list of rape victims is not possible to attain. Rape victims also entered the Convertite in Tuscany; see Cohen, 1988, pp. 64–5.

78. ASV Provveditori sopra Monasteri, Busta 267, "Le Convertide contro Il. Nob. Ho. Tomà Lion et altri nobili," cases begins October 7, 1626 and ends in dismissal January 2, 1627 (m.r.).

79. McGough, 1997, p. 33.

80. ASV Provveditori sopra Monasteri (PsM), Busta 265, fasc. June 22, 1618.

81. ASPV, Archivio Segreto, Visite Pastorali a monastery femminili, Busta 1, fasc. 9, November 20, 1625.

82. ASV PsM, Busta 265, fasc. June 22, 1618, interview with Suor Felice on June 29, 1618.

83. ASV, Sant'Uffizio, Busta 81, Fasc. 2, ff. 27v-28r.

84. Ibid., testimony of Nuntiata, widow of Paolo de Bacchis, August 11, 1626, ff. 13v-14r.

85. Ibid., testimony of Angela Giustiana, f. 30v.

86. Ibid., testimony of Angela Giustiana, September 3. "Ss.ri si. Ne havevo doi casselle; et gli davo da tener dell'acqua et del vin, accio la terra s'ingrassasse, et la herba venisse bella. et dicevo che era buona da farse ben voler, et che venendo bella cresceva l'amor, et che venendo bruta ò morendo, mancava l'amor, ò doveva occorrer qualche cattivo accidente."

87. ASV, Notarile Testamenti, Tes. Chiuso No. 498, Not. Girolamo Brinis, August 21, 1626.

88. M. Barbaro, Vol. IV, p. 18.

89. ASV Sant'Uffizio., Busta 81, fasc. 2, ff. 27v-28r.

90. ASV Provveditori sopra Monasteri, Busta 260, 4 February 1621 m.v.
91. ASV Convertite, Busta 50, Capitoli, f. 7.
92. ASV Provveditori Sopra Monasteri, Busta 260, August 13, 1622.
93. ASV Senato Terra, Register 107, August 3, 1632, ff. 246v-247r.
94. "Parte Pertinente al Povero Hospedal della Pietà et delle Povere Convertide," in *Parti prese in Consiglio Xm in Pregadi* Vol. II (Turin: Carlo Clausen, 1898), ff. 527v-529r; ASV Senato Terra, Reg., July 12, 1622. The Tuscan Convertite was also financed through a tax on prostitution; see Cohen, 1988, p. 51.
95. ASV Senato Terra, Reg. 99, August 5, 1628, f. 219v.
96. ASV Convertite, Busta 70, Fasc. "Notatorio Primo," May 6, 1630, f. 15r.
97. ASV Convertite, Busta 70, Fasc. "Notatorio Primo," September 4, 1646, f. 23v.
98. ASV Convertite, Busta 75, "Parte prese nell'Eccellentiss. Senato 1646. A di 6 Aprile."
99. ASV Convertite, Busta 1, Fasc. D, ff. 5r-6r.
100. ASV Convertite, Busta 70, Fasc. Notatorio Primo, f. 5v-7v.
101. ASV Convertite, Busta 54, loose paper, January 28, 1597 m.v.
102. ASPV, Archivio Segreto, Atti patriarcali riguardanti le monache, March 15, 1599, f. 111v.
103. ASVaticano, Sacra Congregatione, Episcoporum et Reg., Positiones, 1601 Lett. S-V, Urbino (undated).
104. ASVaticano, Sacra Congregatione, Episcoporum et Reg., Positiones, 1651 January–April, in bundle dated January 13, 1651, Bologna.
105. Entrance records are in ASV Convertite, Busta 1, Fasc. D, ff. 5r-6r. and Busta 70, Fasc. Notatorio Primo.
106. Davis, 1991, pp. 3–5; on dowries, see p. 101 and footnote no. 53 on p. 232.
107. Spiritual dowries could run as high as 3000–4000 ducats at the most exclusive convents. See Sperling, 1999, p. 190.
108. Quoted and translated by Cohen, 1988, p. 63.
109. On Naples, see ASVaticano, Sacra Cong., Episcoporum et Regularum, Positiones, 1650 March–July, bundle dated March 24, 1650, letter from Naples. On Ferrara and Gubbio, see 1650 March–July, bundle dated June 4, 1650, Ferrara; 1648 January–June A-V, bundle dated June 26, 1648, Gubbio.
110. Data compiled from ASV Convertite, Busta 1, Fasc. D. The "raised from the devil's jaws" category includes the women coming directly from the Casa del Soccorso. For more on these data, see McGough, 1997, pp. 70–3.
111. ASPV, Archivio Segreto, Visite Pastorali a monasteri femminili, Busta 1, fasc. 9, November 20, 1625.
112. The Patriarch's criticisms were repeated in successive visits. See ASPV, Archivio Segreto, Visite Pastorali a monastery femminili, Busta 1, April 22, 1599, f. 114r; Busta 1, fasc. 9, November 20, 1635, no. 6; Busta 3, January 11, 1593, ff. 82v-83r.
113. McGough, 2002, pp. 32–52.
114. Laven, 2003, pp. 3–8, 23–44.
115. Chojnacka, 1998, p. 82. The beneficiaries of charity were often the "deserving poor" throughout the Italian peninsula. See Pullan, 1971; for Bologna, see Ciammitti, 1979, p. 470.
116. Groppi, 1994, pp. 32–5.
117. Archivio IRE, PEN A1, *Capitoli per il buon governo del pio loco in ovvegno delle povere peccatrici penitentidi San Job* (Venice, 1731).

118. *Capitoli per il buon Governo del Pio Loco in Sovvegno delle Povere Peccatrici Penitentidi San Job* (Venice, 1731), Archivio IRE, PEN A1; Giuliana Marcolini, "Up Epilogo Settecentesco: Le Penitenti di San Job," in *Nel Regno dei Poveri: Arte e Storia dei Grandi Ospedali Veneziani in Età Moderna 1474–1797* (Venezia, IRE 1989).

119. Siena, 2004, p. 214.

120. ASV PSO, Busta 76, fasc. "Ammalati," October 31, 1793 and fasc. 19.

121. Pullan, 1999, pp. 18–39, on p. 19.

122. Cavallo, 1995, p. 228.

123. A useful approach to understanding the complex intellectual, economic, and political background underlying changing attitudes toward poverty during the eighteenth century is Lindemann, 1990, esp. pp. 74–99.

124. *Capitoli per il buon Governo del Pio Loco in Sovvegno delle Povere Peccatrici Penitenti di San Job*, Cap. XXVI. "che siano povere, e così miserabili, che non abbino modo di vivere senza peccare. E però s'escludono le Meretrici bene stanti, e quelle ch'anno arte onesta per procacciarsi il vitto, e quelle che hanno parenti, o persone pie, che possano, e vogliano ajutarle, ed in somma tutte quelle che possono in altra maniera salvarsi."

125. Cavallo, 1995, pp. 254–5.

126. Ferrante, 1990.

127. Musitano, 1871, pp. 13–14. "Ma è falso, ch'il seme si putrefaccia per lo troppo uso di Venere, perche questa peste senza contaggio si sarebbe generata; essendo, ch'il continuo, e li'immoderato uso di Venere fù da che il Mondo era bambino, principalmente doppo quella feconda benedizione: Crescite multiplicamini, replete terram."

128. Musitano, 1871, p. 15. "I soldati Francesi ricevettero le Meretrici, e perche costoro non si vergognano in publico usare, cominciarono à negoziare le Meretrici, & belle, e brutte con gran empito di libidine."

129. Conner, 1996, pp. 15–33, on p. 19.

130. Conner, 1996, p. 24.

131. *Capitoli per il buon Governo del Pio Loco in Sovvegno delle Povere Peccatrici Penitenti di San Job*, Cap. XXVI.

132. *Capitoli per il buon Governo del Pio Loco in Sovvegno delle Povere Peccatrici Penitenti di San Job*, Cap. XXVI, April 26, 1726. "che restino di nuova incaricati li Signori Presidenti andar molto cauti nel proporre alla Congregazione Supplicanti per esser accettatte, senza che prima abbino le più possibile informazioni della loro salute intorno i mali, che sogliono le misere montraere nella prostituzione de' loro Corpi, ed in caso, dopo che fossero accettate, scoprissero detti mali di difficile curazione, assicurati che siano dal Medico, e Chirurgo di un tale stato di alcuna debbano immediatemente, & irremissibilmente licenziarla."

133. *Capitoli per il buon Governo del Pio Loco in Sovvegno delle Povere Peccatrici Penitenti di San Job*, Cap. XXVI.

134. Archivio IRE PEN, G11, November 21, 1730.

135. The trial against Domenico De Silvestro can be found in ASV, Esecutori contro la Bestemmia, Busta 46, June 19, 1793. See testimony of June 20 for explanation of the family's circumstances. A surgeon, Antonio Previdi, examined Lucia and concluded that she had lost her virginity and become infected with the French disease.

136. See testimony of June 22–23 and record of medical inspection of Domenico on June 25. On eighteenth-century cases of sexual relations with children, see Larry Wolff, "'Depraved Inclinations': Libertines and Children in Casanova's Venice," *Eighteenth-Century Studies* 38: 3 (2005), 417–40.

137. On Lucia's treatment with the hospital of the Incurabili, see ASV, Prov. alla Sanità, Busta 76, Fasc. "Ammalati."

138. Braunstein, 1998.

139. Ellero, 1990.

140. Archivio IRE, PEN A1, *Capitoli per il buon Governo del Pio Loco in Sovvegno delle Povere Peccatrici Penitenti di San Job.*

141. *Capitoli per il buon Governo del Pio Loco in Sovvegno delle Povere Peccatrici Penitenti di San Job*, Cap. XXVI, April 26, 1726 addendum. "Che restino di nuova incaricati li Signori Presidenti andar molto cauti nel proporre alla Congregazione Supplicanti per esser accettatte, senza che prima abbino le più possibile informazioni della loro salute intorno i mali, che sogliono le misere montraere nella prostituzione de' loro Corpi, ed in caso, dopo che fossero accettate, scoprissero detti mali di difficile curazione, assicurati che siano dal Medico, e Chirurgo di un tale stato di alcuna debbano immediatemente, & irremissibilmente licenziarla, ne sia sotto alcun preteso lecito trattenerla nella Pia Casa, ed esclusa una volta non possa poi esser proposta per esser di nuovo accettata; anzi per decoro dell'Istituto ne meno possa esser mandata all'Incurabili in avvenire veruna delle Penitenti, ne essere dispensato da questa parte, senza esser proposta alla Congregazione ridotta al numero di 18. con li cinque sesti, e previa la lettura di tutte le parti a questo proposito disponenti."

142. Merians, 2004, pp. 30–61.

143. See especially Harrington, 1999, pp. 308–45; Ogilvie, 2006, pp. 38–78.

144. Berco, 2005, pp. 331–58.

145. Foucault, 1995. For assessments of Foucault's impact, see Jones and Porter, 1994.

146. Useful scholarship using the concept of social disciplining includes Po-Chia Hsia, 1989 and Prodi, 1994.

147. McGough, 2002. Gavitt, 1997, pp. 230–70; Cavallo, 1995; on the financial strategies of charitable institution, see Safley, 1997.

Conclusion

1. ASV, Guidice Petizion, Terminazioni, reg. 133, November 18, 1616, f. 154.

2. Siena, 2004, pp. 254–5.

3. Cohen, 2008, pp. 512–19, on p. 518.

4. Iliffe, 2006, pp. 15–16.

5. Qualtiere and Slights, 2003, pp. 1–24; Harris, 1998.

Afterword

1. Kumeh, 2009, p. 7.

2. Iliffe, 2006, pp. 23, 82, 92.

3. Peter Geshiere even argues that belief in witchcraft should be seen as essentially modern (Geschiere, 1997). As Jean Allman and John Parker point out, however, it is difficult to know whether belief has increased without any reliable measure of the extent of witchcraft belief or accusations in the pre-colonial period. Allman and Parker, *Tongnaab* 2005, p. 116.

4. Thomas, 2007, pp. 279–91; Ashforth, 2002, pp. 121–43.

5. Ashforth, 2002.

6. For how to collaborate with traditional healers and religious leaders, see UNAIDS, 2007; Green, 2000, pp. 1–2; Ssali et al., 2005, pp. 485–93.

7. Sontag, 1977, p. 3.

8. Brown, Macintyre, and Trujillo, 2003, pp. 49–69.

9. AIDS stigma has been identified as one of the principal obstacles to HIV testing worldwide, as well as an obstacle to seeking treatment until patients have reached an advanced stage of disease, often with CD4 cell counts at 50 or below. Patients are usually advised to begin antiretroviral therapy when they reach a CD4 cell count of between 200 and 350. CD4 cell counts of below 50 indicate advanced disease. Valdiserri, 2002, pp. 341–2; UNAIDS, April 2004.

10. Parker and Aggleton, 2003, pp. 13–24.

11. Castle, 2004, p. 11.

12. Sarah Castle, p. 15.

13. Nyblade, et al., 2003.

14. A useful model could be the town hall meetings that have been used to develop health care priorities. These meetings are dialogues between local communities and public health officials, in which the public provides input for the establishment of priorities and provides feedback on official documents. See Daniels and Sabin, 2002. Another model would be to borrow from the literature about conflict resolution and reconciliation, where historical examples from other cultures are used in order to show that conflict is a human problem, not restricted to particular ethnic groups. See Staub, Pearlman, and Miller, 2003, pp. 287–94.

15. Nyblade et al., 2008; Nyblade et al., 2009.

16. Barnett and Whiteside, 2006, pp. 364–9.

17. Schuklenk and Kleinsmidt, 2007, p. 1180.

18. Schulenk and Kleinsmidt, 2007, p. 1182.

19. A notable example of this was the decline in funds for syphilis and gonorrhea control during the 1950s, after the introduction of penicillin for treatment. Entire programs, such as contact tracing, were cut back. Syphilis and gonorrhea rates subsequently rose. See Brandt, 1987, pp. 176–8.

20. Personal communication with Dr. Jonathan Zenilman, Professor of Medicine, Division of Infectious Diseases, Johns Hopkins University School of Medicine, Baltimore, Maryland, July 2005.

21. Stamm, 2008, pp. 575–93, on p. 575.

22. Eng and Butler, 1997, pp. 312–13.

23. Epstein, 2007, p. 76.

24. Pisani, 2008, pp. 134–42.

25. Epstein, 2007, pp. 176–7. The reasons for the decline in Uganda's HIV prevalence stirred up considerable controversy in 2004 and 2005, with

different experts asserting the relative importance of abstinence, condom use, and partner reduction. Epstein was one of the participants in the debate with an emphasis on partner reduction. Epstein's book obviously presents her point of view on this issue on pp. 172–85, with ample footnotes that acknowledge the arguments, scientific studies, and rebuttals presented by her opponents. Pisani (2008) is more even-handed on the issue of Uganda and raises the alarm that, however much HIV prevalence may have declined from the 1980s to the late 1990s, it is unfortunately on the increase again (pp. 144–8).

26. Pisani, 2008, pp. 164–5.

Bibliography

Manuscript Sources

Vatican, Archivio Segreto Vaticano (ASVatican)
  Sacra Congregazione (SC), Episcopourm et Regularium (E & R), Positiones
Venice, Archivio di Stato di Venezia (ASV)
  Convertite
  Provveditori alla Sanità
  Provveditori sopra Monasteri (PSM)
  Provveditori sopra Ospitali (PSO)
  Sant'Uffizio (SU)
Venice, Archivio Storico dell'Istituto di Ricovero e di Educazione (Archivio IRE)
  Zitelle (ZIT)
  Penitenti (PEN)
  Soccorso (SOC)
Venice, Museo Civico Correr (MCC)
  Codice Cicogna 3239

Published Sources

Allen, P. L. (2000) *The Wages of Sin: Sex and Disease, Past and Present* (Chicago: University of Chicago Press).

Allman, J. and Parker, J. (2005) *Tongnaab: The History of a West African God* (Bloomington and Indianapolis: Indiana University Press).

Ambrosini, F. (2000) "Toward a Social History of Women in Venice," in J. Martin and D. Romano (eds.) *Venice Reconsidered: The History and Civilization of an Italian City-State, 1297–1797* (Baltimore: Johns Hopkins University Press).

Ames-Lewis, F. and Rogers, M. (1998) *Concepts of Beauty in Renaissance Art* (Brookfield, VT: Ashgate).

Anarfi, J. K. and Awusabo-Asare, K. (1993) "Experimental Research on Sexual Networking in Some Selected Areas of Ghana," *Health Transition Review* 3, Supplementary Issue, 1–15.

Aretino, P. (1976) *Selected Letters*, G. Bull (transl.) (New York: Penguin).

Arrizabalaga, J. (1994) "Facing the Black Death: Perceptions and Reactions of University Medical Practitioners," in Luis Garcia-Ballester, Roger French, Jon Arrizabalaga, and Andrew Cunningham (eds.) *Practical Medicine from Salerno to the Black Death* (New York, Cambridge: Cambridge University Press), pp. 237–88.

Arrizabalaga, J. (1999) "Medical Causes of Death in Preindustrial Europe: Some Historiographical Considerations," *Journal of the History of Medicine* 54, 241–60.

Arrizabalaga, J. (2005) "Medical Responses to the 'French Disease' in Europe at the Turn of the Sixteenth Century," in K. Siena (ed.) *Sins of the Flesh: Responding to Sexual Disease in Early Modern Europe* (Toronto: Centre for Reformation and Renaissance Studies).

Arrizabalaga, J., Henderson, J. and French, R. (1997) *The Great Pox: The French Disease in Renaissance Europe* (New Haven and London: Yale University Press).

Ashforth, A. (2000) *Madumo: A Man Bewitched* (Chicago: University of Chicago Press).

Ashforth, A. (2002) "An Epidemic of Witchcraft? The Implications of AIDS for the Post-Apartheid State," *African Studies* 61, 121–43.

Badir, P. (1999) "'To allure vntu their loue': Iconoclasm and Striptease in Lewis Wager's *The Life and Repentance of Mary Magdalene*," *Theater Journal* 51, 1–20.

Baker, B. J. and Armelagos, G. J. (1988) "The Origin and Antiquity of Syphilis: Paleopathological Diagnosis and Interpretation," *Current Anthropology* 29, 703–37.

Barlow, D. (2001) "Heterosexual Transmission of HIV-1 Infection in UK," *Lancet* 358 (9291): 1458.

Basaldella, F. (1986) *Giudecca: Storia e testimonianze* (Venice: Marcon Uniongrafica).

Bellavitis, A. (1998) "Dot et Richesse des femmes à Venise au XVIe siècle," *Clio: Histoire, Femmes et Société* 7, 91–100.

Benedetti, A. (1549) *Il fatto d'arme del Tarro fra i principi Italiani, et Carlo Ottavo Re de Francia*, translated from the Latin by Lodovico Domenichi Book 1 (Venice: Gabriel Giolito de Ferrari).

Bennett, S. and Chanfreau, C. (2005) "Approaches to Rationing Antiretroviral Treatment: Ethical and Equity Implications," *Bulletin of the World Health Organization 2005* 83 (7), 541–7.

Berco, C. (2005) "Social Control and Its Limits: Sodomy, Local Sexual Economies, and Inquisitors during Spain's Golden Age," *Sixteenth Century Journal* 36(2), 331–58.

Berco, C. (2007) "Syphilis and the Silencing of Sodomy in Juan Calvo's *Tratado del morbo gálico*," in K. Borris and G. Rousseau (eds.) *The Sciences of Homosexuality in Early Modern Europe* (London: Routledge).

Berkowitz, S. D. (1982) *An Introduction to Structural Analysis: The Network Approach to Social Research* (Toronto: Butterworths).

Bernstein, L. (1995) *Sonia's Daughters: Prostitutes and Their Regulation in Imperial Russia* (Berkeley: University of California Press).

Boily, M. C., Poulin, R. and Mâsse (November 2000) "Some Methodological Issues in the Study of Sexual Networks: From Model to Data to Model," *Sexually Transmitted Diseases* 27, 558–72.

Boschini, M. (1664) *Le Minere della Pittura* (Venice: F. Nicolini).

Bottigheimer, R. B. (2002) *Fairy Godfather: Straparola, Venice, and the Fairy Tale Tradition* (Philadelphia: University of Pennsylvania Press).

Bouwsma, W. J. (1968) *Venice and the Defense of Republican Liberty: Renaissance Values in the Age of the Counter Reformation* (Berkeley, LA: University of California Press).

Brandt, A. (1987) *No Magic Bullet: A Social History of Venereal Disease in the United States since 1880*, 2nd edition (New York, Oxford: Oxford University Press).

Braunstein, P. (1998) "Cannaregio, zona di transito?," in D. Lanaro (ed.) *La città italiana e I luoghi degli stranieri, XIV–XVIII secolo* (Rome: Laterza).

Brockliss, L. and Jones, C. (1997) *The Medical World of Early Modern France* (Oxford: Clarendon Press).

Brown, D. A. (2001) *Virtue and Beauty: Leonardo's Ginevra de' Benci and Renaissance Portraits of Women* (Washington, DC: National Gallery of Art and Princeton: Princeton University Press).

Brown, J. C. and Davis, R. C. (eds.) (1998) *Gender and Society in Renaissance Italy* (New York: Longman).

Brown, L., Macintyre, K. and Trujillo, L. (2003) "Interventions to Reduce HIV/ AIDS Stigma: What Have We Learned?" *AIDS Education and Prevention* 15(1), 49–69.

Brundage, J. (1987) *Law, Sex, and Christian Society in Medieval Europe* (Chicago: University of Chicago Press).

Buehrer, B. T. (1990) "Early Modern Syphilis," *Journal of the History of Sexuality* 1, 197–214.

Bylebyl, J. "The Manifest and the Hidden in the Renaissance Clinic," in W. F. Bynum and R. Porter (eds.) *Medicine and the Five Senses* (Cambridge: Cambridge University Press).

Cady, D. (2005) "Linguistic Dis-ease: Foreign Language as Sexual Disease in Early Modern England," in K. Siena (ed.) *Sins of the Flesh: Responding to Sexual Disease in Early Modern Europe* (Toronto: Centre for Renaissance and Reformation Studies).

Camerano, A. (April 1993) 'Assistenza richiesta ed assistenza imposta: il conservatorio di S. Caterina della Rosa di Roma', *Quaderni Storici* 82, 227–60.

Campbell, C. (2003) *Letting Them Die: Why HIV/AIDS Prevention Programmes Fail* (Bloomington, Indiana and Oxford, UK: Indiana University Press).

Campbell, M. (1992) "Carnal Knowledge: Fracastoro's *De Syphilis* and the Discovery of the New World," in D. Segal (ed.) *Crossing Cultures: Essays in the Displacement of Western Civilization* (Tucson and London: University of Arizona Press).

Capitoli et Ordini per il buon Governo della Congregatione del Monastero di S. Maria Maddalena delle Convertite della Giudecca (Venice: Lovisa, 1719), pp. 8–11.

Carlin, C. L. (ed.) (2005) *Imagining Contagion in Early Modern Europe* (New York: Palgrave Macmillan).

Carlino, A. (1999) "Paper Bodies: A Catalogue of Anatomical Fugitive Sheets 1538–1687," *Medical History Supplement* no. 19 (London: Wellcome Institute for the History of Medicine).

Carmichael, A. (1991) "Syphilis and the Columbian Exchange: Was the Disease Really New?," in M. G. Marques and J. Cule (eds.) *The Great Maritime Discoveries and World Health* (Lisbon: Ecola Nacional de Saúde Pública).

Carmichael, A. (1998) "Epidemics and State Medicine in Fifteenth-Century Milan," in R. French, J. Arrizabalaga, A. Cunningham, and L. García-Ballester (eds.) *Medicine from the Black Death to the French Disease* (Brookfield US: Ashgate).

Carmichael, A. G. (1991) "Contagion Theory and Contagion Practice in Fifteenth-Century Milan," *Renaissance Quarterly* 44, 213–56.

Castle, S. (2004) "Rural Children's Attitudes to People with HIV/AIDS in Mali: The Causes of Stigma," *Culture, Health & Sexuality* 6(1).

Cavallo, J. A. (2004) *The Romance Epics of Boiardo, Ariosto, and Tasso: From Public Duty to Private Pleasure* (Toronto: University of Toronto Press).

Cavallo, S. (1995) *Charity and Power in Early Modern Italy: Benefactors and Their Motives in Turin, 1541–1789* (New York: Cambridge University Press).

Chauncey, G., Duberman, G. and Vicinus, M. (eds.) (1989) *Hidden from History: Reclaiming the Gay and Lesbian Past* (New York: New American Library).

Chojnacka, M. (1998) "Women, Charity and Community in Early Modern Venice: The Casa delle Zitelle," *Renaissance Quarterly* 51, 68–91.

Chojnacka, M. (2001) *Working Women of Early Modern Venice* (Baltimore: Johns Hopkins University Press).

Chojnacka, M. (January 2000) "Women, Men, and Residential Patterns in Early Modern Venice," *Journal of Family History* 25(1), 6–25.

Chojnacki, S. (1975) "Dowries and Kinsmen in Early Modern Venice," *Journal of Interdisciplinary History* 5(4), 571–600.

Chojnacki, S. (1990) "Marriage Legislation and Patrician Society in Fifteenth-Century Venice," in B. Bachrach, D. Nicholas, and B. D. Lyon (eds.) *Law, Custom, and the Social Fabric in Medieval Europe* (Kalamazoo: Western Michigan University Medieval Institute Publications).

Chojnacki, S. (2000) *Women and Men in Renaissance Venice: Twelve Essays on Patrician Society* (Baltimore and London: Johns Hopkins University Press).

Ciammitti, L. (1979) "Conservatori femminili a Bologna e Organizzazione del Lavoro," *Quaderni Storici* 41, 760–4.

Cipolla, C. (1976) *Public Health and the Medical Profession in the Renaissance* (Cambridge: Cambridge University Press).

Cipolla, C. (1981) *Fighting the Plague in Seventeenth-Century Italy* (Madison, WI: University of Wisconsin Press).

Cipolla, C. (1970) "I Libri dei Morti," *Le Fonti della Demografia Storica in Italia* (Rome: CISP) Vol. I, Pt. II, 851–66.

Coates, T. J. (2001) *Convicts and Orphans: Forced and State-Sponsored Colonizers in the Portuguese Empire, 1550–1755* (Stanford: Stanford University Press).

Cochrane, E. (1988) *Italy 1530–1630* (London and New York: Longman).

Cohen, E. S. (1998) "Seen and Known: Prostitutes in the Cityscape of Late-Sixteenth-Century Rome," *Renaissance Studies* 12(3), 392–409.

Cohen, J. (July 2008) "The Great Funding Surge," *Science* 321, 512–19.

Cohen, S. (1992) *The Evolution of Women's Asylums since 1500: From Refuges for Ex-Prostitutes to Shelters for Battered Women* (New York: Oxford University Press).

Cohn, S. (1996) *Women in the Streets: Essays on Sex and Power in Renaissance Italy* (Baltimore: Johns Hopkins University Press).

Conner, S. P. (1996) "The Pox in Eighteenth-Century France," in L. E. Merians (ed.) *The Secret Malady: Venereal Disease in Eighteenth-Century Britain and France* (Lexington: University Press of Kentucky).

Corbin, A. (1990) *Women for Hire: Prostitution and Sexuality in France after 1850*, A. Sheridan (transl.) (Cambridge, MA: Harvard University Press).

Corradi, A. (Milan 1871) "Nuovi Documenti per la storia delle malattie veneree in Italia della fine del '400 alla metà del '500," *Rendiconti* 4, 14–15, 1–32.

Coryat, T. (1611) *Coryats Crudities*, 2nd edition (London: William Stansby).

Cowan, A. (1999) 'Patricians and Partners in Early Modern Venice,' in E. Kittell and T. Madden (eds.) *Medieval and Renaissance Venice* (Urbana and Chicago: University of Illinois Press).

Cox, V. (1995) "The Single Sex: Feminist Thought and the Marriage Market in Early Modern Venice," *Renaissance Quarterly* 48: 3, 513–81.

Crawford, K. (June 2006) "Privilege, Possibility, and Perversion: Rethinking the Study of Early Modern Sexuality," *The Journal of Modern History* 78, 412–33.

Creytens, R. (1965) "La riforma dei monastery femminili dopo i decreti tridentini," in *Concilio di Trento e la riforma tridentina*, vol. 1 Atti del convegno storico
internazionale (Rome: Herder).

Crosby, A. W. (1972) *The Columbian Exchange: Biological and Social Consequences
of 1492* (Westport, CT: Greenwood Press).

Cunningham, A. (2002) "Transforming Plague: The Laboratory and the
Identity of Infectious Disease," in A. Cunningham and P. Williams (eds.)
The Laboratory Revolution in Medicine (Cambridge, UK: Cambridge University
Press).

Dabhoiwala, F. (2001) "Sex, Social Relations and the Law in Seventeenth- and
Eighteenth-Century London," in M. J. Braddick and J. Walter (eds.) *Negotiating
Power in Early Modern Society: Order, Hierarchy and Subordination in Britain and
Ireland* (Cambridge: CUP), pp. 85–101.

Daniels, N. and Sabin, J. E. (2002) *Setting Limits Fairly: Can We Learn to Share
Medical Resources* (New York: Oxford University Press).

Daston, L. and Park, K. (2001) *Wonders and the Order of Nature, 1150–1750* (New
York: Zone Books).

Davidson, N. S. (2002) "Sodomy in Early Modern Venice," in T. Betteridge (ed.)
Sodomy in Early Modern Europe (Manchester: Manchester University Press).

Davis, G. (2008) *"The Cruel Madness of Love": Sex, Syphilis and Psychiatry in
Scotland, 1880–1930* (Amsterdam, New York: Rodopi).

Davis, J. (1975) *A Venetian Family and Its Fortune, 1500–1900: The Donà and the
Conservation of their Wealth* (Philadelphia: American Philosophical Society).

Davis, N. Z. (1987) *Fiction in the Archives: Pardon Tales and Their Tellers in Sixteenth-
Century France* (Stanford: Stanford University Press).

Davis, R. C. (1991) *Shipbuilders of the Venetian Arsenal: Workers and Workplace in
the Preindustrial City* (Baltimore: Johns Hopkins University Press).

Davis, R. C. (1994) *The War of the Fists: Popular Culture and Public Violence in Late
Renaissance Venice* (Oxford: Oxford University Press).

De morbo gallico omnia quae extant apud omnes medicos cujuscunque nationis
(1566–7) (Venice: Jordanum Zilettum).

de Renzi, S. (1999) "'A Fountain for the Thirsty' and a Bank for the Pope: Charity,
Conflicts, and Medical Careers at the Hospital of Santo Spirito in Seventeenth-
Century Rome," in Ole Peter Grell, Andrew Cunningham, Jon Arrizabalaga
(eds.) *Health Care and Poor Relief in Counter-Reformation Europe* (New York:
Routledge).

Della Porta, G. (1598) *Della fisonomia dell'huomo* (Naples: Tarquinio Longo).

Douglas, M. (1966) *Purity and Danger: An Analysis of the Concepts of Pollution and
Taboo* (London: Routledge and Kegan Paul).

Dumont, D. (1998) "Women and Guilds in Bologna: The Ambiguities of
'Marginality," *Radical History Review* 70, 4–25.

Eamon, W. (1998) "Cannibalism and Contagion: Framing Syphilis in Counter-
Reformation Italy," *Early Science and Medicine* 3(1), 1–31.

Eamon, W. (1994) *Science and the Secrets of Nature: Books of Secrets in Medieval and
Early Modern Culture* (Princeton: Princeton University Press).

Eatough, G. (ed. and transl.) (1984) *Fracastoro's Syphilis* (Liverpool: Francis
Cairns).

Eglin, J. (2001) *Venice Transfigured: The Myth of Venice in British Culture, 1660–
1797* (New York: Palgrave Macmillan).

Eisenach, E. (2004) "Husbands, Wives, and Concubines: Marriage, Family, and Social Order in Sixteenth-Century Verona," *Sixteenth Century Essays & Studies* 69 (Kirksville, MO: Truman State University Press).

Ellero, G. (1990). "I Luoghi della Redenzione," in *Le Cortigiane di Venezia dal Trecento al Settecento* (Venice: Berenice).

Eng, T. R and Butler, W. T (1997) *The Hidden Epidemic: Confronting Sexually Transmitted Diseases* (Washington, DC: National Academy Press).

Epstein, H. (2007) *The Invisible Cure: Why We are Losing the Fight against AIDS in Africa* (New York: Picador/Farrar, Straus and Giroux).

Estienne, C. (1546) *La Dissection des parties du corps* (Paris: Simon de Colines).

Fairchilds, C. (1984) *Domestic Enemies: Servants and Their Masters in Old Regime France* (Baltimore: Johns Hopkins University Press).

Farmer, P. (1992) *AIDS and Accusation: Haiti and the Geography of Blame* (Berkeley: University of California Press).

Favero, G., Moro, M., Spinelli, P., Trivellato, F. and Vianello, F. (1991) "Le anime dei demografi: Fonti per la rivelazione dello stato della popolazione di Venezia nei secoli XVI e XVII," *Bolletino di Demografia Storica* 15, 23–110.

Ferrante, L. (1986) "Pro mercede carnali ... Il giusto prezzo rivendicato in tribunale," *Memoria* 17(2), 51–3.

Ferrante, L. (1990) "Honor Regained: Women in the Casa del Soccorso di San Polo in Sixteenth-Century Bologna" in E. Muir and G. Ruggiero (eds.) *Sex and Gender in Historical Perspective* (Baltimore: Johns Hopkins University Press).

Ferraro, J. (2001) *Marriage Wars in Late Renaissance Venice* (Oxford: Oxford University Press).

Ferro, M. (1845) *Dizionario del Diritto Comune e Veneto* (Venice: Andrea Santini e Figlio).

Findlen, P. (1993) "Humanism, Politics, and Pornography in Renaissance Italy," in L. Hunt (ed.) *The Invention of Pornography: Obscenity and the Origins of Modernity, 1500–1800* (New York: Zone Books).

Fitzgerald, A. (1988) *Conversion through Penance in the Italian Church of the Fourth and Fifth Centuries: New Approaches to the Experience of Conversion from Sin*, Studies in the Bible and Early Christianity, 15 (Lewiston, NY: The Edwin Mellen Press).

Foa, A. (1990) "The New and the Old: The Spread of Syphilis (1494–1530)," in Edward Muir and Guido Ruggiero (eds.) *Sex and Gender in Historical Perspective* (Baltimore: Johns Hopkins University Press).

Fonte, M. (Modesta Pozzo) (1997) *The Worth of Women: Wherein is Clearly Revealed Their Nobility and Their Superiority to Men*, Virginia Cox (ed. and transl.) (Chicago: University of Chicago Press).

Foucault, M (1995) *Discipline and Punish: The Birth of the Prison*, A. Sheridan (transl.), 2nd edition (New York: Vintage Books).

Freedberg, D. (1989) *The Power of Images: Studies in the History and Theory of Response* (Chicago: University of Chicago Press).

Frelick, N. (2005) "Contagions of Love: Textual Transmission," in Claire Carlin (ed.) *Imagining Contagion in Early Modern Europe*, pp. 47–62.

French, R. and Arrizabalaga, J. (1998) "Coping with the French Disease: University Practitioners' Strategies and Tactics in the Transition from the Fifteenth to the Sixteenth Century," in R. French, J. Arrizabalaga, A. Cunningham, and L. García-Ballester (eds.) *Medicine from the Black Death to the French Disease* (Brookfield, VT: Ashgate).

Gallucci, M. A. (2003) *Benvenuto Cellini: Sexuality, Masculinity, and Artistic Identity in Renaissance Italy* (New York: Palgrave Macmillan).

Gambacini, P. (2004) *Mountebanks and Medicasters: A History of Italian Charlatans from the Middle Ages to the Present*, B. G. Lippitt (transl.) (Jefferson, NC: McFarland).

Gambier, M. (1980) "La Donna e la giustizia penale veneziana nel XVII secolo," in G, Cozzi (ed.) *Stato, Società e Giustizia nella Repubblica Veneta (Sec. XV–XVIII)* (Rome: Jouvence).

Gavitt, P. (June 1997) "Charity and State Building in Cinquecento Florence: Vincenzo Borghini as Administrator of the Ospedale degli Innocenti," *Journal of Modern History* 69, 230–70.

Gemin, M. (1990) "Le cortigiane di Venezia e i viaggiatori stranieri," in D. D. Poli and I. Ariano (eds.) *Il gioco dell'amore: Le Cortigiane di Venezia dal trecento al settecento* (Milan: Berenice).

Gentilcore, D. (1998) *Healers and Healing in Early Modern Italy* (Manchester: Manchester University Press).

Gentilcore, D. (2005) "Charlatans, the Regulated Marketplace and the Treatment of Venereal disease in Italy," in K. Siena (ed.) *Sins of the Flesh: Responding to Sexual Disease in Early Modern Europe* (Toronto: Centre for Reformation and Renaissance Studies).

Gentilcore, D. (2006) *Medical Charlatanism in Early Modern Italy* (Oxford, New York: Oxford University Press).

Gevitz, N. (2000) "The Devil Hath Laughed at the Physicians," *Journal of the History of Medicine* 55, 5–36.

Gibson, M. (1986) *Prostitution and the State in Italy, 1860–1915* (Columbus, OH: Ohio State University Press).

Gilman, S. (1993) "Touch, Sexuality and Disease," in W. F. Bynum and R. Porter (eds.) *Medicine and the Five Senses* (Cambridge: Cambridge University Press).

Glass, T. A. and McAtee, M. J. (2006) "Behavioral Science at the Crossroads in Public Health: Extending Horizons, Envisioning the Future," *Social Science & Medicine* 62, 1650–71.

Goffen, R. (1997) *Titian's Women* (New Haven and London: Yale University Press).

Goffman, E. (1963) *Stigma: Notes on the Management of a Spoiled Identity* (New York: Simon and Schuster).

Gras, M. J., Weide, M. W., Coutinho, R. A., and van den Hoek, A. (1999) "HIV Prevalence, Sexual Risk Behaviour and Sexual Mixing Patterns among Migrants in Amsterdam, the Netherlands," *AIDS* 13, 1953–62.

Green, E. C. (2000) "Traditional Healers and AIDS in Uganda," *The Journal of Alternative and Complementary Medicine* 6, 1–2.

Grendler, P. (1977) *The Roman Inquisition and the Venetian Press, 1540–1605* (Princeton: Princeton University Press).

Griffin, G. (2000) *Representations of HIV and AIDS: Visibility Blue/s* (Manchester: Manchester University Press).

Groppi, A. (1994) *I Conservatori della Virtù: Donne Recluse nella Roma dei Papi* (Rome: Laterza).

Grubb, J. (1986) "When Myths Lose Power: Four Decades of Venetian Historiography," *Journal of Modern History* 58(1), 43–94.

Hacke, D. (2004) *Women, Sex and Marriage in Early Modern Venice* (Burlington, VT: Ashgate).

Hanlon, G. (1998) *The Twilight of a Military Tradition: Italian Aristocrats and European Conflicts, 1560–1800* (New York: Holmes & Meier).

Harper, K. N., Ocampo, P. S., Steiner, B. M., George, R. W., Silverman, M. S., Bolotin, S., Pillay, A., Saunders, N. J., and Armelagos, G. J. (2008) "On the Origin of Treponematoses: A Phylogenetic Approach," *PLoS Negl Trop Dis* 2(1), 148.

Harrington, J. F. (1999) "Escape from the Great Confinement: The Genealogy of a German Workhouse," *Journal of Modern History* 71, 308–45.

Harris, J. G. (1998) *Foreign Bodies and the Body Politic: Discourses of Social Pathology in Early Modern England* (Cambridge, UK: Cambridge University Press).

Harris, J. G. (2004) *Sick Economies: Drama, Mercantilism and Disease in Shakespeare's England* (Philadelphia: University of Pennsylvania Press).

Haskins, S. (1993) *Mary Magdalene: Myth and Metaphor* (New York: Harcourt Brace).

Hay, D. and Law, J. (1989) *Italy in the Age of the Renaissance, 1380–1530* (London and New York: Longman).

Healy, M. (2001) *Fictions of Disease in Early Modern England: Bodies, Plagues and Politics* (New York: Palgrave Macmillan).

Henderson, J. (2006) *The Renaissance Hospital: Healing the Body and Healing the Soul* (New Haven and London: Yale University Press).

Henderson, J. (1999) "Charity and Welfare in Early Modern Tuscany," in O. P. Grell, A. Cunningham, and J. Arrizabalaga (eds.) *Health Care and Poor Relief in Counter-Reformation Europe* (New York: Routledge).

Hentschell, R. (2005) "Luxury and Lechery: Hunting the French Pox in Early Modern England," in K. Siena (ed.) *Sins of the Flesh: Responding to Sexual Disease in Early Modern Europe* (Toronto: Centre for Renaissance and Reformation Studies).

Hewlett, M. (2005) "The French Connection: Syphilis and Sodomy in Late-Renaissance Lucca," in K. Siena (ed.) *Sins of the Flesh: Responding to Sexual Disease in Early Modern Europe* (Toronto: Centre for Renaissance and Reformation Studies).

Horodowich, L. (2005) "Armchair Travelers and the Venetian Discovery of the New World," *Sixteenth Century Journal* XXXVI/4: 1031–62.

Hyde, S. T. (2007) *Eating Spring Rice: The Cultural Politics of AIDS in Southwest China* (Berkeley, LA: University of California Press).

Iliffe, J. (2006) *The African AIDS Epidemic: A History* (Oxford, UK and Athens, Ohio: James Currey and Ohio University Press).

Jones, C. and Porter, C. (eds.) (1994) *Reassessing Foucault: Power, Medicine, and the Body* (New York: Cambridge University Press).

Karras, R. M. (1996) *Common Women: Prostitution and Sexuality in Medieval England* (New York: Oxford University Press).

Katritzky, M. A. (2001) "Marketing Medicine: The Image of the Early Modern Mountebank," *Renaissance Studies* 15(2): 121–253.

Kent, F. W. and Simons, P. (1987) *Patronage, Art and Society in Renaissance Italy* (Oxford: Clarendon Press).

Kirshner, J. (1978) *Pursuing Honor While Avoiding Sin: The Monte delle doti of Florence* (Milan: A. Giuffrè).

Kisacky, J. M. (2000) *Magic in Boiardo and Ariosto* (New York: Peter Lang).

Klapisch-Zuber, C. (1985) *Women, Family and Ritual in Renaissance Italy*, L. Cochrane (transl) (Chicago: University of Chicago Press).

Klovdahl, A. S. (1985) "Social Networks and the Spread of Infectious Diseases: The AIDS Example," *Social Science & Medicine* 21(11), 1203–16.

Kuehn, T. (1991) *Law, Family, and Women: Toward a Legal Anthropology of Renaissance Italy* (Chicago: University of Chicago Press).

Kumeh, T. (2009) "My Pastor said He'd Healed Me of HIV," *The Ghanaian Times.* September 16, 2009, p. 7.

Kunze, M. (1987) *Highroad to the Stake: A Tale of Witchcraft,* W. Yuill (transl.) (Chicago: University of Chicago Press).

Lachmund, J. and Stollberg, G. (eds.) (1992) *The Social Construction of Illness: Illness and Medical Knowledge in Past and Present* (Stuttgart: Franz Steiner).

Lane, F. C. (1973) *Venice: A Maritime Republic* (Baltimore: Johns Hopkins University Press).

Lansing, C. (2003) "Concubines, Lovers, Prostitutes: Infamy and Female Identity in Medieval Bologna," in P. Findlen, M. M. Fontaine, and D. J. Osheim (eds.) *Beyond Florence: The Contours of Medieval and Early Modern Italy* (Stanford: Stanford University Press).

Larivaille, P. (1980) *Pietro Aretino fra Rinascimento e Manierismo,* M. di Maio and M. L. Rispoli (transl.) (Rome: Bulzoni).

Laughran, M. (1998) *The Body, Public Health, and Social Control in Sixteenth-Century Venice* (PhD Dissertation, University of Connecticut).

Laughran, M. (October, 2002) "Regulating Bodies: Public Health and Social Control in Sixteenth-Century Venice," paper presented at "The Body in Early Modern Italy" conference (Johns Hopkins University, Baltimore, MD).

Laughran, M. A. (2003) "Oltre la pelle. I cosmetici e il loro uso," in Carlo Marco Belfanti and Fabio Giusberti (eds.) *Storia d'Italia* Annali 19 *La moda* (Turin: Einaudi).

Laven, M. (2003) *Virgins of Venice: Broken Vows and Cloistered Lives in the Renaissance Convent* (New York: Viking).

Lawner, L. (1989) *I Modi: The Sixteen Pleasures: An Erotic Album of the Italian Renaissance* (Evanston, IL: Northwestern University Press).

Leavitt, J. (1996) *Typhoid Mary: Captive to the Public's Health* (Boston: Beacon Press).

Levack, B. P. (1995) *The Witch-Hunt in Early Modern Europe,* 2nd edition (New York: Longman).

Liebowitz, R. (1979) "Virgins in the Service of Christ: The Dispute over an Active Apostolate for Women during the Counter-Reformation," in R. Ruether and E. McLaughlin (eds.) *Women of Spirit: Female Leadership in the Jewish and Christian Traditions* (New York: Simon and Shuster).

Lindemann, M. (1990) *Patriots and Paupers: Hamburg, 1712–1830* (New York, Oxford: Oxford University Press).

Lindemann, M. (1999/2006) *Medicine and Society in Early Modern Europe* (New York and Cambridge: Cambridge University Press).

Link, B. G. and Phelan, J. C. (2001) "Conceptualizing Stigma," *Annual Review of Sociology* 27, 363–85.

Lobera, Luigi (1558) *Libro delle Quattro Infermita Cortigiane* (Venice: Gio. Battista & Marchio Sessa).

Lualdi, K. J. and Thayer, A. T. (eds.) (2000) *Penitence in the Age of Reformations* (Burlington, VT: Ashgate).

Lurie, M. N., Williams, B. G., Zuma, K., Mkaya-Mwamburi, D., Garnett, G. P., Sweat, M. D., Gittelsohn, J., and Karim, S. S. (2003) "Who Infects Whom?

HIV-1 Concordance and Discordance among Migrant and Non-Migrant Couples in South Africa," *AIDS* 17, 2245–52.

Lurie, M. N., Williams, B. G., Zuma, K., Mkaya-Mwamburi, D., Garnett, G. P., Sturm, A. W., Sweat, M. D., Gittelsohn, J., and Abdool Karim, S. S. (2003) "The Impact of Migration on HIV-1 Transmission in South Africa: A Study of Migrant and Nonmigrant Men and Their Partners," *Sexually Transmitted Diseases* 30, 149–56.

Mackenney, R. (1987) *Tradesmen and Traders: The World of the Guilds in Venice and Europe, c. 1250–c. 1650* (London: Croom Helm).

Maclean, I. (1980) *The Renaissance Notion of Woman* (New York, Cambridge: Cambridge University Press).

Maclean, I. (1999) "The Notion of Woman in Medicine, Anatomy, and Physiology," in L. Hutson (ed.) *Feminism and Renaissance Studies* (Oxford: Oxford University Press).

Mallett, M. E. (1974) *Mercenaries and Their Masters: Warfare in Renaissance Italy* (Totoaw, NJ: Rowman and Littlefield).

Mallett, M. E. (1984) *The Military Organization of a Renaissance State: Venice c. 1400 to 1617* (Cambridge: Cambridge University Press).

Malvern, M. M. (1975) *Venus in Sackcloth: The Magdalen's Origins and Metamorphoses* (Carbondale: Southern Illinois University Press).

Marinello, G. (1574) *Gli Ornamenti delle Donne* (Venice: Giovanni Valgrifio).

Marques, M. G. and Cule, J. (eds.) (1991) *The Great Maritime Discoveries and World Health* (Lisbon: Escola National de Saúde Pública, Ordem dos Médicos, Instituto de Sintra).

Martin, J. (1993) *Venice's Hidden Enemies: Italian Heretics in a Renaissance City* (Berkeley: University of California Press).

Martin, J. and Romano, D. (eds.) (2000) *The History and Civilization of an Italian City-State, 1297–1797* (Baltimore: Johns Hopkins University Press).

Martin, R. (1989) *Witchcraft and the Inquisition in Venice, 1550–1650* (New York: Basil Blackwell).

Martini, G. (1986–7) "La Donna Veneziana del '600 tra Sessualità Legittima ed Illegittima: Alcune Reflessioni sul Concubinato," *Atti dell'Istituto Veneto di Scienze, Lettere ed Arti*, CXLV, 305–26.

Massa, N. (1566) *Il Libro del Mal Francese* (Venice: Giordano Ziletti).

Maza, S. (1983) *Servants and Masters in Eighteenth-Century France: The Uses of Loyalty* (Princeton: Princeton University Press).

McGough, L. J. (2006) "Demons, Nature or God? Witchcraft Accusations and the French Disease in Early Modern Venice," *Bulletin of the History of Medicine* 80(2), 219–46.

McGough, L. J. (2005) "Quarantining Beauty: The French Disease in Early Modern Venice," in K. Siena (ed.) *Sins of the Flesh: Responding to Sexual Disease in Early Modern Europe* (Toronto: Centre for Reformation and Renaissance Studies), pp. 211–37.

McGough, L. J. (1997) "Raised from the Devil's Jaws": A Convent for Repentant Prostitutes in Venice, 1530–1670 (PhD dissertation, Northwestern University).

McGough, L. J. (2002) "Women, Private Property, and the Limitations of State Authority in Early Modern Venice," *Journal of Women's History*, 14(3), 32–52.

McGough, L. and Erbelding, E. (2006) "Historical Evidence of Syphilis and Other Treponemes," in S. Lukehart and J. Radolf (eds.) *Pathogenic Treponema: Molecular and Cellular Biology* (Norfolk, England: Horizon Scientific Press/ Caister Academic Press), pp. 183–95.

McGough, L. J., Reynolds, S. J., Quinn, T. C., and Zenilman, J. M. (July 2005) "Which Patients First? Setting Priorities for Antiretroviral Therapy Where Resources are Limited," *American Journal of Public Health* 95(7), 1173–80.

McNeill, W. (1972). *The Columbian Exchange: Biological and Cultural Consequences of 1492* (Westport, CT: Greenwood Press).

McNeill, W. (1998 edition; original 1976) *Plagues and Peoples* (New York: Anchor books).

Menghi, G. (1605; original edition 1576) *Compendio dell'arte essorcista* (Venice: Giovanni Varisco).

Mercurio, G. S. (1658) *Degli Errori Popolari d'Italia* (Padova: Matteo Cadorino).

Mercurio, G. S. (1621) *La Commare Oriccoglitrice* (Venice: Giovanni Battista Ciotti).

Molà, L. (2000) *The Silk Industry of Renaissance Venice* (Baltimore: Johns Hopkins University Press).

Molho, A. (1979) "Cosimo de Medici: Pater Patriae or Padrino?," *Stanford Italian Review* 1, 5–33.

Molho, A. (1988) "Patronage and the State in Early Modern Italy," *Klientelsysteme im Europa der Frühen Neuzeit* (Munich: Verlag).

Molmenti, P. (1906) *La Storia di Venezia nella Vita Privata*, Vol. II (Bergamo: Istituto Italiano d'arti grafiche).

Monter, E. W. (1990) *The Frontiers of Heresy: The Spanish Inquisition from the Basque Lands to Sicily* (Cambridge: Cambridge University Press).

Monter, E. W. (1976) *Witchcraft in France and Switzerland: The Borderlands during the Reformation* (Ithaca: Cornell University Press).

Montrose, L. (1991) "The Work of Gender in the Discourse of Discovery," *Representations* No. 33, Special Issue: The New World.

Morris, M., Goodreau, S. and Moody, J. (2008) "Sexual Networks, Concurrency, and STD/HIV," in K. K. Homes, F. P. Sparling, W. E. Stamm, P. Piot, J. N. Wasserheit, L. Corey, M. S. Cohen, and D. H. Watts (eds.) *Sexually Transmitted Diseases*, 4th edition (New York: McGraw Hill).

Mosco, M. (1986) *La Maddalena tra sacro e profano: da Giotto a De Chirico* (Florence: Casa Usher).

Muir, E. (1981) *Civic Ritual in Renaissance Venice* (Princeton: Princeton University Press).

Muir, E. (1991) "Observing Trifles," in E. Muir and G. Ruggiero (eds.) *Microhistory and the Lost Peoples of Europe* (Baltimore: Johns Hopkins University Press).

Muir, E. (2007) *The Culture Wars of the Late Renaissance: Skeptics, Libertines, and Opera* (Cambridge: Harvard University Press).

Muir, E. and Ruggiero, G. (eds.) (1994) *History from Crime* (Baltimore: Johns Hopkins University Press).

Mulligan, C. J., Norris, S. J., Lukehart, S. J. (2008) 'Molecular Studies in *treponema pallidum* Evolution: Toward larity?," *PLoS Negl Trop Dis* 2(1), 184.

Musa Brasavola, Antonio. (1553) *Examen omnium Loch; idest linctuum, suffuf, idest pulverum, aquarum, decoctionum, oleorum, quorum apud Ferrarienses pharmacopolas usus est, ubi De morbo Gallico...* (Venice: Apud Juntas).

Nguyen, V. K., Grennan, T., Peschard, K., Tan, D., and Tiendrebeogo, I. (2003) "Antiretroviral Use in Ougadougou, Burkina Faso," *AIDS* 17, Supplement 3, S109–S111.

Nordio, A. (1993/4) *Tra Carità e sanità. La nascita degli Incurabili nella Venezia del primo '500*, Tesi di Laurea (Venice: University of Venice).

Nordio, A. (1996) "L'Ospedale degli Incurabili nell'Assistenza Veneziana del '500," *Studi veneziani* N.S., XXXII, 170.

Nordio, A. (1994) "Presenze Femminili nella Nascita dell'Ospedale degli Incurabili di Venezia," *Regnum Dei* 120, 11–17.

Nutton, V. (1983) "The Seeds of Disease: An Explanation of Contagion and Infection from the Greeks to the Renaissance," *Medical History* 27, 1–34.

O'Malley, J. (1993) *The First Jesuits* (Cambridge: Harvard University Press).

O'Neil, M. (1987) "Magical Healing, Love Magic and the Inquisition in Late Sixteenth-Century Modena," in S. Haliczer (ed.) *Inquisition and Society in Early Modern Europe* (London: Croom Helm).

O'Neil, M. R. (1984) "*Sacerdote ovvero strione*: Ecclesiastical and Superstitious Remedies in 16th Century Italy," in S. L. Kaplan (ed.) *Understanding Popular Culture: Europe from the Middle Ages to the Nineteenth Century* (New York: Mouton Publishers).

Ogilvie, S. (January 2006) "'So That Every Subject Knows How to Behave': Social Disciplining in Early Modern Bohemia," *Comparative Studies in Society and History* 48(01), 38–78.

Opera Nova Intitolata Dificio de Recette nella quale si contengono tre utilissimi recettari (Venice, 1530).

Opera Nuova Intitolata Dificio di Ricette, nella quale si contengono tre utilissimi ricettari (Venice, 1526).

Ostetriche (Secoli XVI–XIX) (Milan: Franco Angeli, 1984).

Otis, L. L. (1985) *Prostitution in Medieval Society: The History of an Urban Institution in Languedoc* (Chicago: University of Chicago Press).

Pallucchini, R. (1981) *La Pittura Veneziana del Seicento* (Milan: Electa).

Palmer, R. (1978) The Control of Plague in Venice and Northern Italy, 1348–1600 (PhD Thesis, University of Kent).

Palmer, R. (1983) *The Studio of Venice and Its Graduates in the Sixteenth Century* (Center for the History of the University of Padua, Trieste: Edizioni Lint).

Palmer, R. (1985) "Pharmacy in the Republic of Venice in the Sixteenth Century," in A. Wear, R. French, and I. Lonie (eds.) *The Medical Renaissance of the Sixteenth Century* (Cambridge: Cambridge University Press).

Palmer, R. (1999) "Ad Una Sancta Perfettione': Health Care and Poor Relief in the Republic of Venice in the Era of the Counter-Reformation," in O. P. Grell, A. Cunningham, J. Arrizabalaga (eds.) *Health Care and Poor Relief in Counter-Reformation Europe* (New York: Routledge).

Pancino, C. (1984) *Il Bambino e L'Acqua Sporca: Storia dell'Assistenza al Parto dale Mammane* (Milan: Franco Angeli).

Pancino, C. (2003) "*Soffrire per ben comparire. Corpo e bellezza, natura e cura*," in C. M. Belfani and F. Giusberti (eds.) *Storia d'Italia*, Annali 19 *La moda* (Turin: Einaudi).

Paré, A. (1982) *On Monsters and Marvels*, J. L. Pallister (transl.) (Chicago: University of Chicago Press).

Parker, R. and Aggleton, P. (2003) "HIV and AIDS-Related Stigma and Discrimination: A Conceptual Framework and Implications for Action," *Social Science & Medicine* 57, 15–26.

"Parte Pertinente al Povero Hospedal della Pietà et delle Convertide," in *Parti prese in Consiglio Xm in Pregadi* Vol. II (Turin: Carlo Clausen, 1898).

Pavan, E. (1980) "Police des moeurs, société et politique à Venise à la fin du Moyen Age," *Revue historique* 268, 241–88.

Pelling, M. (2003) *Medical Conflicts in Early Modern London* (Oxford: Clarendon Press).

Pisani, E. (2008) *The Wisdom of Whores: Bureaucrats, Brothels and the Business of AIDS* (London: Granta).

Po-Chia Hsia, R. (1989) *Social Discipline in the Reformation: Central Europe 1550–1750* (London and New York: Routledge).

Poirer, G. (2005) "A Contagion at the Source of Discourse on Sexualities: Syphilis during the French Renaissance," in C. L. Carlin (ed.) *Imagining Contagion in Early Modern Europe* (New York: Palgrave Macmillan).

Pomata, G. (1999) "Practicing between Earth and Heaven: Women Healers in Seventeenth-Century Bologna," *Dynamis* 19, 119–43.

Pomata, G. (1998) *Contracting a Cure: Patients, Healers, and the Law in Early Modern Bologna* (Baltimore: Johns Hopkins University Press).

Porter, R. (1997) *The Greatest Benefit to Mankind: A Medical History of Humanity* (New York: Norton).

Porter, R. (2000) *Quacks: Fakers and Charlatans in English Medicine* (Charleston, SC: Tempest).

Porter, R. and Rousseau, G. C. (1998) *Gout: The Patrician Malady* (New Haven: Yale University Press).

Preto, P. (1978) *Peste e società a Venezia nel 1576* (Vicenza: Pozzi).

Prodi, P. (1994) *Disciplina dell'anima, disciplina del corpo e disciplina della società fra Medioevo ed Età Moderna* (Bologna: Il Mulino).

Pullan, B. (1999) "The Counter-Reformation, Medical Care and Poor Relief," in O. P. Grell, A. Cunningham, and J. Arrizabalaga (eds.) *Health Care and Poor Relief in Counter-Reformation Europe* (New York: Routledge).

Pullan, B. (1971) *Rich and Poor in Renaissance Venice: The Social Institutions of a Catholic State* (Oxford: Blackwell).

Puppi, L. (1994) *Le Zitelle: architettura, arte e storia di un'istituzione veneziana* (Venice: Albrizzi).

Qualtiere, L. F. and Slights, W. W. E. (2003) "Contagion and Blame in Early Modern England: The Case of the French Pox," *Literature and Medicine* 22(1), 1–23.

Quétel, C. (1990) *History of Syphilis* (Baltimore: Johns Hopkins University Press).

Ranger, T. and Slack, P. (eds.) (1996) *Epidemics and Ideas: Essays on the Historical Perception of Pestilence*, 2nd edition (New York, Cambridge: Cambridge University Press).

Rocke, M. (1995) "Gender and Sexual Culture in Renaissance Italy," in J. Brown and R. Davis (eds.) (1998) *Gender and Society in Renaissance Italy* (New York: Longman).

Rocke, M. (1996) *Forbidden Friendships: Homosexuality and Male Culture in Renaissance Florence* (Oxford: Oxford University Press).

Rogers, M. (1988) "The Decorum of Women's Beauty: Trissino, Firenzuola, Luigini and the Representation of Women in Sixteenth-Century Painting," *Renaissance Studies* 2(1), 47–87.

Rollo-Koster, J. (2002) "From Prostitutes to Brides of Christ: The Avignonese *Repenties* in the late Middle Ages," *Journal of Medieval and Early Modern Studies* 32(1), 109–44.

Romano, D. (1996) *Housecraft and Statecraft: Domestic Service in Renaissance Venice 1400–1600* (Baltimore: Johns Hopkins University Press).

Romano, D. (1987) *Patricians and Popolani: The Social Foundations of the Venetian Renaissance State* (Baltimore: Johns Hopkins University Press).

Romano, D. (1989) "Gender and the Urban Geography of Renaissance Venice," *Journal of Social History* 23(2), 339–54.

Roper, L. (1985) "Discipline and Respectability: Prostitution and the Reformation in Augsburg," *History Workshop Journal* 21(19), 3–28.

Rosaldo, R. (1986) "From the Door of His Tent: The Fieldworker and the Inquisitor," in J. Clifford and G. Marcus (eds.) *Writing Culture: The Poetics and Politics of Ethnography* (Berkeley: University of California Press).

Rosen, S., Senne, A., Collier, A., and Simon, J. (2005) "Hard Choices: Rationing Antiretroviral Therapy for HIV/AIDS in Africa," *The Lancet 2005* 365(9456), 354–6.

Rosenberg, C. and Golden, J. (eds.) (1992) *Framing Disease: Studies in Cultural History* (New Brunswick, NJ: Rutgers University Press).

Rosenthal, M. (1992) *The Honest Courtesan: Veronica Franco, Citizen and Writer in Sixteenth-Century Venice* (Chicago: University of Chicago Press).

Rossiaud, J. (1988) *Medieval Prostitution*, L. Cochrane (transl.) (Cambridge, MA: Blackwell).

Rostinio, P. (transl. of Musa Brasavola's *De Morbo Gallico*) (1556, reprint 1559) *Trattato del mal francese* (Venice: Lodovico Avanzi).

Rostinio, P. (transl. of Musa Brasavola's *De Morbo Gallico*) (1565) *Trattato del mal francese* (Venice: Giorgio de' Cavalli).

Ruether, R. and McLaughlin, E. (eds.) (1979) *Women of Spirit: Female Leadership in the Jewish and Christian Traditions* (New York: Simon and Shuster).

Ruggerio, G. (1993) "Marriage, Love, Sex, and Renaissance Civic Morality," in James Grantham Turner (ed.) *Sexuality and Gender in Early Modern Europe: Institutions, Texts, Images* (Cambridge: Cambridge University Press).

Ruggiero, G. (1985) *The Boundaries of Eros: Sex Crime and Sexuality in Renaissance Venice* (Oxford: Oxford University Press).

Ruggiero, G. (1993) *Binding Passions: Tales of Magic, Marriage and Power at the End of the Renaissance* (New York: Oxford University Press).

Ruggiero, G. (2001) "The Strange Death of Margarita Marcellini: Male, Signs, and the Everyday World of Pre-Modern Medicine," *American Historical Review* 106(4), 1141–58.

Ruggiero, G. (April 1978) "The Cooperation of Physicians and the State in the Control of Violence in Renaissance Venice," *Journal of the History of Medicine*, 156–84.

Safley, T. M. (1997) *Charity and Economy in the Orphanages of Early Modern Augsburg* (Atlantic Highlands, NJ: Humanities Press).

Sansovino, F. (1581) *Venetia Città Nobilissima et Singolare* (Venice: Jacopo Sansovino).

Sanuto, Marino (1878–1903) *I Diarii di Marin Sanuto*, ed. Rinaldo Fulin, 58 vols. (Venice: F. Visentini).

Schleiner, W. (1994) "Infection and Cure through Women: Renaissance Constructions of the French Disease," *Journal of Medieval and Renaissance Studies* 24(3), 499–517.

Schleiner, W. (1994) "Moral Attitudes toward Syphilis and Its Prevention in the Renaissance," *Bulletin of the History of Medicine* 68, 389–410.

Schuler, C. M. (1991) "The Courtesan in Art: Historical Fact or Modern Fantasy?," *Women's Studies* 19, 209–22.

Schutte, A. J. (2001) *Aspiring Saints: Pretence of Holiness, Inquisition, and Gender in the Republic of Venice, 1618–1750* (Baltimore: Johns Hopkins University Press).

Scott, J. (1991) *Social Network Analysis: A Handbook* (Newbury Park, CA: Sage Publications).

Secreti Diversi & miracolosi (Venice: Alessandro Gardano, 1578), pp. 28–43.

Shemek, D. (2004) *Medusa's Gaze: Essays on Gender, Literature, and Aesthetics in the Italian Renaissance. In Honor of Robert J. Rodini,* Paul A. Ferrara, Eugenio Giusti and Jane Tylus (eds.). Italiana XI (Boca Raton, Florida: Bordighera Press), pp. 49–64.

Shilts, R. (1987) *And the Band Played On: People, Politics, and the AIDS Epidemic* (New York: St. Martin's Press).

Siena, K. (2001) "The Foul Disease' and Privacy: The Effects of Venereal Disease and Patient Demand in the Medical Marketplace in Early Modern London," *Bulletin of the History of Medicine* 75, 199–224.

Siena, K. (2007) "The Strange Medical Silence on Same-Sex Transmission of the Pox, c. 1660–c. 1760," in K. Borris and G. Rousseau (eds.) *The Sciences of Homosexuality in Early Modern Europe* (London: Routledge).

Siena, K. P. (2004) *Venereal Disease, Hospitals, and the Urban Poor: London's "Foul Wards," 1600–1800* (Rochester: University of Rochester Press).

Siraisi, N. G. (1997) *The Clock and the Mirror: Girolamo Cardano and Renaissance Medicine* (Princeton: Princeton University Press).

Sontag, S. (1977) *Illness as Metaphor* (New York: Vintage Books).

Sperling, J. (1999) *Convents and the Body Politic in Late Renaissance Venice* (Chicago: University of Chicago Press).

Spongberg, M. (1997) *Feminizing Venereal Disease: The Body of the Prostitute in Nineteenth-Century Medical Discourse* (New York: New York University Press).

Ssali, A., Butler, L. M., Kabetsi, D., King, R., Namugenyi, A., Kamya, M. R., Mandel, J., Chen, S. Y., and McFarland, S. W. (2005) "Traditional Healers for HIV/AIDS Prevention and Family Planning, Kiboge District, Uganda: Evaluation of a Program to Improve Practices," *AIDS and Behavior* 9, 485–93.

Stamm, W. E. (2008) "*Chlamydia trachomatis* Infections of the Adult," in K. K. Homes, F. P. Sparling, W. E. Stamm, P. Piot, J. N. Wasserheit, L. Corey, M. S. Cohen, and D. H. Watts (eds.), *Sexually Transmitted Diseases*, 4th edition (New York: McGraw-Hill).

Staub, E., Pearlman, L. A., and Miller, V. (2003) "Healing the Roots of Genocide in Rwanda," *Peace Review* 15(3), 287–94.

Steele, B. (1997) "In the Flower of Their Youth: 'Portraits' of Venetian Beauties ca. 1500," *Sixteenth Century Journal* 28(2), 481–502.

Stein, C. (2006) "The Meaning of Signs: Diagnosing the French Pox in Early Modern Augsburg," in *Bulletin of the History of Medicine* 80, 617–47.

Tedeschi, J. (1991) *The Prosecution of Heresy: Collected Studies on the Inquisition in Early Modern Italy* (Binghamton, NY: Center for Medieval and Early Renaissance Studies).

Thomas, F. (2007) "'Our Families are Killing Us': HIV/AIDS, Witchcraft, and Social Tensions in the Caprivi Region, Namibia," *Anthropology and Medicine* 14, 279–91.

Tramontin, S. (1972) "Lo spirito, le attività, gli svilluppi dell'oratorio del Divino Amore nella Venezia del Cinquecento," *Studi veneziani* XIV, 111–36.

Treichler, P. A. (1988) "AIDS, Gender, and Biomedical Discourse: Current Contests for Meaning," in E. Fee and D. M. Fox (eds.) *AIDS: The Burdens of History* (Berkeley: University of California Press).

Trivellato, F. (1998) "Out of Women's Hands: Notes on Venetian Glass Beads, Female Labour and International Trades," in L. Sciama and J. Eicher (eds.) *Beads and Bead Makers: Gender, Material Culture and Meaning* (New York: Berg).

UNAIDS (2007) *Collaborating with Traditional Healers for HIV Prevention and Care in Sub-Saharan Africa: Suggestions for Programme Managers and Field Workers* (Geneva, Switzerland).

UNAIDS (April 2004) *Stepping Back from the Edge: The Pursuit of Antiretroviral Therapy in Botswana, South Africa, and Uganda* (Geneva).

Valdiserri, R. O. (March 2002) "HIV/AIDS Stigma: An Impediment to Public Health," *American Journal of Public Health* 93(3).

van Deusen, N. E. (2001) *Between the Sacred and the Worldly: The Institutional and Cultural Practice of Recogimiento in Colonial Lima* (Stanford: Stanford University Press).

Voltaire (1990) *Candide* (Oxford: Oxford University Press).

Wailoo, K. (2001) *Dying in the City of Blues: Sickle Cell Anemia and the Politics of Race and Health* (Chapel Hill: University of North Carolina Press).

Walker, J. (1998) "Bravi and Venetian Nobles, c. 1550–1650," *Studi veneziani* 26, 100.

Walkowitz, J. (1980) *Prostitution and Victorian Society: Women, Class, and the State* (New York: Cambridge University Press).

Watkins, S. C. (1995) "Social Networks and Social Science History," *Social Science History* 19, 295–311.

Weaver, E. B. (2003) "A Reading of the Interlaced Plot of the *Orlando Furioso*: The Three Cases of Love Madness," in D. Beecher, M. Ciavolella, and R. Fedi (eds.) *Ariosto Today: Contemporary Perspectives* (Toronto: University of Toronto Press).

Weinstein, D. (1970) *Savonarola and Florence: Prophecy and Patriotism in the Renaissance* (Princeton, NJ: Princeton University Press).

Wellman, B. and Wetherell, B. (1996) "Social Network Analysis of Historical Communities: Some Questions form the Past," *History of the Family* 1, 97–121.

Wetherell, C. (1998) "Historical Social Network Analysis," *International Review of Social History* 43, supplement 6, 125–44.

Wetherell, C. (Spring1989) "Network Analysis Comes of Age," *Journal of Interdisciplinary History* XIX, 645–51.

Wetherell, C., Plakans, A., and Wellman, B. (Spring 1994) "Social Networks, Kinship, and Community in Eastern Europe," *Journal of Interdisciplinary History* XXIV, 645.

Wilson, B. (2005) *The World in Venice: Print, the City, and Early Modern Identity* (Toronto: University of Toronto Press).

Wolff, L. (2005) "Depraved Inclinations': Libertines and Children in Casanova's Venice," *Eighteenth-Century Studies* 38(3), 417–40.

Yavneh, N. (1993) "The Ambiguity of Beauty in Tasso and Petrarch," in J. G. Turner (ed.) *Sexuality and Gender in Early Modern Europe: Institutions, Texts, Images* (Cambridge: Cambridge University Press).

Zago, R. (1982) *I Nicolotti: Storia di una Communità I Pescatori a Venezia nell'Età Moderna* (Padua: Francisci).

Zanré, D. (2005) "French Diseases and Italian Responses: Representations of the Mal Francese in the Literature of Cinquecento Tuscany," in K. Siena (ed.) *Sins of the Flesh* (Toronto: Centre for Renaissance and Reformation Studies).

Index